Objective Structured Practical Examination in Physiology

Objective Structured Practical Examination in Physiology

Aarti Sood Mahajan MBBS MD
Professor, Department of Physiology
Maulana Azad Medical College
New Delhi, India

JAYPEE BROTHERS MEDICAL PUBLISHERS (P) LTD
St Louis (USA) • Panama City (Panama) • New Delhi • Ahmedabad • Bengaluru
Chennai • Hyderabad • Kochi • Kolkata • Lucknow • Mumbai • Nagpur

Published by
Jitendar P Vij
Jaypee Brothers Medical Publishers (P) Ltd

Corporate Office
4838/24 Ansari Road, Daryaganj, **New Delhi** 110 002, India, +91-11-43574357
Fax: +91-11-43574314

Registered Office
B-3 EMCA House, 23/23B Ansari Road, Daryaganj, **New Delhi** 110 002, India
Phones: +91-11-23272143, +91-11-23272703, +91-11-23282021
+91-11-23245672, Rel: +91-11-32558559 Fax: +91-11-23276490, +91-11-23245683
e-mail: jaypee@jaypeebrothers.com, Website: www.jaypeebrothers.com

Branches

- 2/B, Akruti Society, Jodhpur Gam Road Satellite
  Ahmedabad 380 015   Phones: +91-79-26926233,   Rel: +91-79-32988717
  Fax: +91-79-26927094   e-mail: ahmedabad@jaypeebrothers.com

- 202 Batavia Chambers, 8 Kumara Krupa Road, Kumara Park East
  Bengaluru 560 001   Phones: +91-80-22285971, +91-80-22382956
  +91-80-22372664,   Rel: +91-80-32714073
  Fax: +91-80-22281761   e-mail: bangalore@jaypeebrothers.com

- 282 IIIrd Floor, Khaleel Shirazi Estate, Fountain Plaza, Pantheon Road
  Chennai 600 008   Phones: +91-44-28193265, +91-44-28194897
  Rel: +91-44-32972089 Fax: +91-44-28193231   e-mail: chennai@jaypeebrothers.com

- 4-2-1067/1-3, 1st Floor, Balaji Building, Ramkote Cross Road
  Hyderabad 500 095   Phones: +91-40-66610020
  +91-40-24758498, Rel:+91-40-32940929
  Fax:+91-40-24758499,   e-mail: hyderabad@jaypeebrothers.com

- No. 41/3098, B & B1, Kuruvi Building, St. Vincent Road
  Kochi 682 018, Kerala   Phones: +91-484-4036109, +91-484-2395739
  +91-484-2395740 e-mail: kochi@jaypeebrothers.com

- 1-A Indian Mirror Street, Wellington Square
  Kolkata 700 013   Phones: +91-33-22651926, +91-33-22276404, +91-33-22276415
  Fax: +91-33-22656075   e-mail: kolkata@jaypeebrothers.com

- Lekhraj Market III, B-2, Sector-4, Faizabad Road, Indira Nagar
  Lucknow 226 016   Phones: +91-522-3040553, +91-522-3040554
  e-mail: lucknow@jaypeebrothers.com

- 106 Amit Industrial Estate, 61 Dr SS Rao Road, Near MGM Hospital, Parel
  Mumbai 400012   Phones: +91-22-24124863, +91-22-24104532
  Rel: +91-22-32926896 Fax: +91-22-24160828,   e-mail: mumbai@jaypeebrothers.com

- "KAMALPUSHPA" 38, Reshimbag, Opp. Mohota Science College, Umred Road
  Nagpur 440 009 (MS)   Phone: Rel: +91-712-3245220
  Fax: +91-712-2704275   e-mail: nagpur@jaypeebrothers.com

North America Office
1745, Pheasant Run Drive, Maryland Heights (Missouri), MO 63043, USA   Ph: 001-636-6279734
e-mail: jaypee@jaypeebrothers.com, anjulav@jaypeebrothers.com

Central America Office
Jaypee-Highlights Medical Publishers Inc., City of Knowledge, Bld. 237, Clayton, Panama City, Panama   Ph: 507-317-0160

Objective Structured Practical Examination in Physiology

© 2010, Jaypee Brothers Medical Publishers

All rights reserved. No part of this publication should be reproduced, stored in a retrieval system, or transmitted in any form or by any means: electronic, mechanical, photocopying, recording, or otherwise, without the prior written permission of the author and the publisher.

> This book has been published in good faith that the material provided by author is original. Every effort is made to ensure accuracy of material, but the publisher, printer and author will not be held responsible for any inadvertent error(s). In case of any dispute, all legal matters are to be settled under Delhi jurisdiction only.

First Edition: **2010**
ISBN: 978-81-8448-786-2
Typeset at   JPBMP typesetting unit
Printed at   Rajkamal Electric Press, Plot No. 2, Phase-IV, Kundli, Haryana

To

**My Parents
and
My Daughters**

Preface

OSPE or Objective Structured Practical Examination is a form of assessment to supplement and decrease the shortfalls of a conventional examination. It may, however, in time to come, replace the conventional examination. Important criteria like objectivity, validity, reliability and practicability are the points in favor for this form of evaluation.

Two types of questions are generally included. These are the question station and the procedure station. In procedure station, the student is asked to perform a small procedure, for which a checklist is already prepared and given to the examiner. It tells the examiner what to expect from the students. If the step is attempted by the student, it is ticked in the checklist by the examiner. Marks are allocated for each step according to importance. In this book checklist is prepared from the examiner's view. For question station, 2 to 3 short questions with definite answers are included. In this book, some questions seem to be repeated in order to show how different combinations may be made in the time frame allotted. The procedure stations test the psychomotor skills. Question stations may test cognitive domain. However, they can be formulated to include the affective domain, especially those testing clinical skills using real or simulated patients.

This book is divided into four units, i.e. hematology, amphibian experiments, mammalian experiments and human experiments. These form the basis of any practical examination in physiology. It includes commonly asked questions. In course of time, new questions will be added. This book could be useful for MBBS, MD, BDS and DNB students. Although the questions pertain to physiology, but the book may be useful for students of pathology, pharmacology and medicine. Some answers are given in the end of the book.

General principles of OSPE include:
1. Divide the entire practical into smaller units or stations
2. Allocate time and marks for each
3. Validate the questions regularly.

Aarti Sood Mahajan

Contents

UNIT 1: HEMATOLOGY

1. Study of Compound Microscope 3
2. Collection of Blood Sample 5
3. Determining of Specific Gravity of Blood 7
4. Estimation of Hemoglobin 8
5. Estimation of Red Blood Cell (RBC) Count 10
6. Estimation of RBC Indices 13
7. Determining of Osmotic Fragility of the RBC 14
8. Determining of Erythrocyte Sedimentation Rate (ESR) and Packed Cell Volume (PCV) 16
9. Estimation of Blood Groups 19
10. Determination of Reticulocyte Count 21
11. Estimation of Total Leukocyte Count 23
12. Preparation of a Smear and Differential Leukocyte Count 25
13. Determining of Absolute Eosinophil Count 28
14. Determination of Bleeding and Clotting Time 30
15. Determination of Platelet Count 32
16. Study of Bone Marrow 34

UNIT 2: AMPHIBIAN EXPERIMENTS

17. Experimental Set-up and Simple Muscle Twitch 37
18. Effect of Temperature on the Simple Muscle Twitch 39
19. Effect of Two Successive Stimuli on Skeletal Muscle Contraction 40
20. Effect of Increasing Strength of Stimulus on Skeletal Muscle Contraction 42
21. Effect of Increasing Frequency of Stimulus on Skeletal Muscle Contraction 43
22. After Loaded and Free Loaded Condition 46
23. Genesis of Fatigue in Skeletal Muscle 49
24. Recording of Isometric Contraction 51
25. Determination of Conduction Velocity of the Sciatic Nerve ... 52
26. Recording of Normal Cardiogram and Effect of Temperature on Normal Cardiogram 54
27. Properties of the Cardiac Muscle 56
28. Effect of Stimulation of the Vagus Nerve and White Crescentic Line on the Cardiogram 59
29. Effect of Some Variables on the Isolated Frog's Heart and the Intact Frog's Heart 61

UNIT 3: MAMMALIAN EXPERIMENTS

30. Effect of Drugs on Movements of Small Intestine of Rabbit 65
31. Effect of Drugs and Variables on Perfusion of Isolated Heart of Rabbit 66

UNIT 4: HUMAN EXPERIMENTS

32. Demonstration of Fatigue using Mosso's Ergograph 71
33. Recording of Systemic Arterial Blood Pressure 73
34. Effect of Posture on Blood Pressure 76
35. Effect of Exercise on Blood Pressure 77
36. Measurement of Blood Flow using Venous Occlusion Plethysmography 79
37. Recording of ECG 81
38. Effect of Exercise on Cardiovascular System 83
39. Study of Respiratory Movements by Stethography 84
40. Study of Lung Function by Spirometry 87
41. Effect of Posture on Vital Capacity 89
42. Effect of Exercise on the Respiratory System 90
43. Measurement of Basal Metabolic Rate 91
44. Determination of Mechanical Efficiency 92
45. Cardiopulmonary Resuscitation 93
46. Recording of Normal Body Temperature and Effect of Hot and
    Cold Environment on It 94
47. Semen Analysis 96
48. Pregnancy Diagnostic Tests 98
49. General Physical Examination 99
50. Clinical Examination of the Cardiovascular System 103
51. Clinical Examination of the Respiratory System 108
52. Clinical Examination of the Abdomen 110
53. Clinical Examination of the Sensory System 114
54. Clinical Examination of the Visual Acuity 118
55. Clinical Examination of Color Vision 120
56. Clinical Examination of the Eye by Retinoscopy and Ophthalmoscopy 121
57. Examination of Field of Vision by Perimetry 122
58. Clinical Examination of Cranial Nerve 124
59. Clinical Examination of Hearing 128
60. Clinical Examination of the Motor System 131
61. Clinical Examination of Higher Functions 135
62. Clinical Examination of Reflexes 136
63. Determination of Reaction Time 139
64. Electroencephalography 141
65. Evoked Potentials 143
    Answers 147
    Index *177*

Unit 1

Hematology

1. Study of Compound Microscope
2. Collection of Blood Sample
3. Determining of Specific Gravity of Blood
4. Estimation of Hemoglobin
5. Estimation of Red Blood Cell (RBC) Count
6. Estimation of RBC Indices
7. Determining of Osmotic Fragility of the RBC
8. Determining of Erythrocyte Sedimentation Rate (ESR) and Packed Cell Volume (PCV)
9. Estimation of Blood Groups
10. Determination of Reticulocyte Count
11. Estimation of Total Leukocyte Count
12. Preparation of a Smear and Differential Leukocyte Count
13. Determining of Absolute Eosinophil Count
14. Determination of Bleeding and Clotting Time
15. Determination of Platelet Count
16. Study of Bone Marrow

Chapter 1

Study of Compound Microscope

PROCEDURE STATION-1

Focus the microscope as you would like to examine the slide in low power.

Checklist

1. Puts the slide on the stage.
2. Cleans the eyepiece.
3. Brings the object on the central aperture of the stage.
4. Focuses the light on the object by adjusting the plain mirror.
5. Partially closes the diaphragm.
6. Lowers the 10X objective on the slide.
7. Puts the condenser to the low position.
8. Looks into the eyepiece and raises the optical tube using coarse adjustment.
9. Brings the slide into focus using fine adjustment.

PROCEDURE STATION-2

Focus the microscope as you would like to examine the slide in high power.

Checklist

1. Puts the slide on the stage.
2. Cleans the eyepiece
3. Brings the object on the central aperture of the stage.
4. Focuses the light on the object by adjusting the concave mirror.
5. The diaphragm. is fully opened
6. Lowers the 40X objective on the slide.
7. Puts the condenser to the middle position.
8. Looks into the eyepiece and raises the optical tube using coarse and fine adjustment.

PROCEDURE STATION-3

Focus the microscope as you would like to examine the slide in oil immersion.

Checklist

1. Puts the slide on the stage.
2. Puts a drop of cedar wood oil on the slide.
3. Cleans the eyepiece.
4. Brings the object on the central aperture of the stage.
5. The diaphragm is fully opened.
6. Places the 100X objective on the slide.
7. Puts the condenser to the top position.
8. Lowers the optical tube so that the lower end dips into the oil.
9. Looks into the eyepiece and raises the optical tube using fine adjustment.

QUESTION STATION

1. Identify the instrument.
2. Identify marked parts of the microscope.
3. Name two types of microscopes that can be used to visualize human tissue.
4. What is the magnification produced by:
   a. High power
   b. Oil immersion lens power.
5. In which power is maximum light made available?

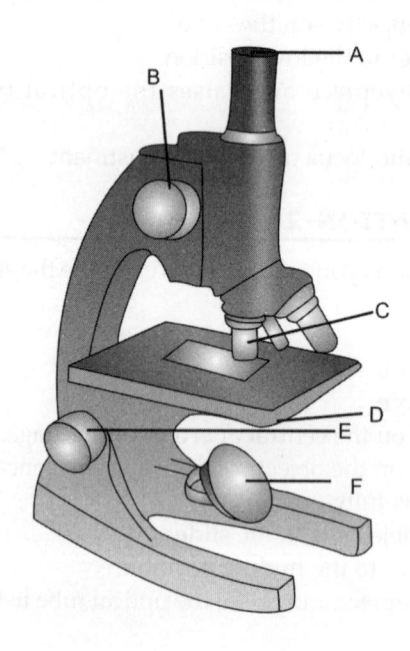

Chapter 2

Collection of Blood Sample

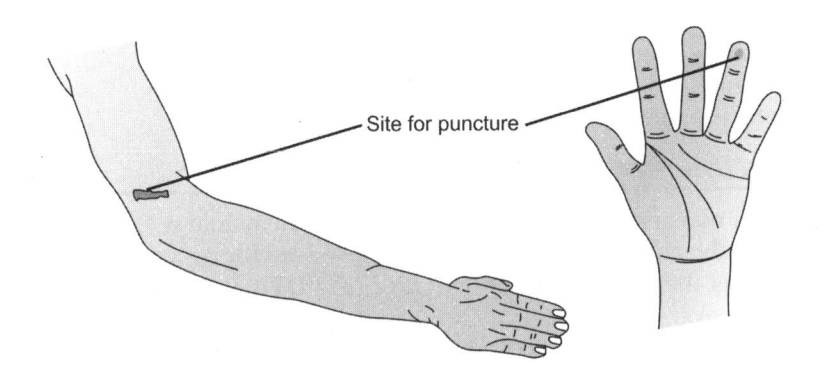

Site for puncture

PROCEDURE STATION-1

Demonstrate how you would collect a venous blood sample.

Checklist

1. Instructs the subject.
2. Wears gloves.
3. Exposes the vein.
4. Cleans the skin over the area with spirit.
5. Allows the spirit to dry.
6. Chooses a disposable syringe.
7. Chooses a disposable needle.
8. Fixes the needle on the syringe.
9. Puts a tourniquet on the subjects arm.
10. Fixes the vein with one hand.
11. Places the needle with its tip at an angle below the vein.
12. Makes the needle enter the vein.
13. The piston of the syringe is gradually withdrawn.
14. Loosens the tourniquet.
15. Collects the required amount of blood.
16. Takes out the needle.

17. Firmly presses the insertion point with a cotton swab.
18. Quickly transfers the collected blood to the collection container/tube.

PROCEDURE STATION-2

Demonstrate the procedure of pricking the finger.

Checklist

1. Instructs the subject.
2. Wears gloves.
3. Chooses the digital third or fourth finger.
4. Cleans the palmer surface of the skin on the finger with spirit.
5. Allows the spirit to dry.
6. Pricks the finger 3-5 mm away from the nail bed.
7. The prick is 3-5 mm deep.
8. There is a free flow of blood.

QUESTION STATION

1. Name two anticoagulants routinely used in hematology experiments.
2. Name the anticoagulant which can be used *in vitro* as well as *in vivo*.
3. What is the mechanism of action of (a) EDTA (b) Trisodium citrate (c) Heparin.
4. What precautions would you take while taking a blood sample?
5. Name two diseases that can spread by improper handling of the blood sample.

Chapter 3
Determining of Specific Gravity of Blood

QUESTION STATION

1. Test tubes containing copper sulphate solution of specific gravity ranging from 1.050 to 1.066 are placed in front of you.

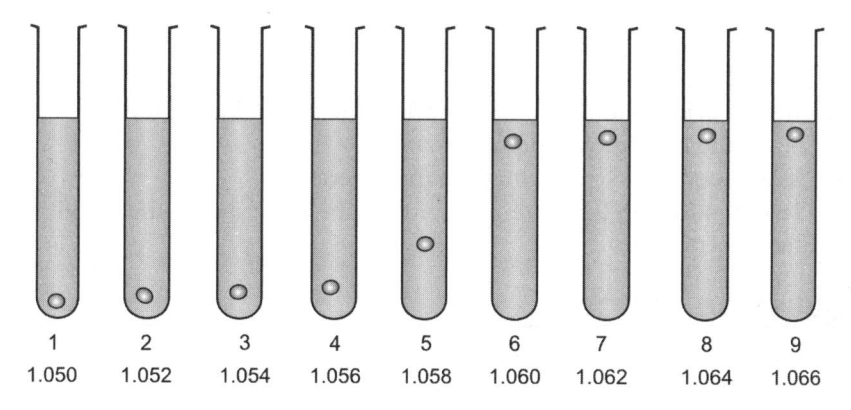

1	2	3	4	5	6	7	8	9
1.050	1.052	1.054	1.056	1.058	1.060	1.062	1.064	1.066

   a. What is the specific gravity of blood?
   b. Why does the drop of blood sink in tube 1?
   c. Why does the drop of blood float in tube 8?
   d. Name one other method used for calculating the specific gravity of blood.
   e. What is the importance of knowing the specific gravity of blood?

2. The diagram shows the procedure for measuring the specific gravity of blood
   a. What is the specific gravity observed?
   b. Is it within normal limit?
   c. Name two conditions in which the specific gravity of the blood is altered?

3. The specific gravity of blood was found to be 1.000
   a. Is it within normal limit?
   b. Name one method of estimating the specific gravity of blood.
   c. What is the importance of estimating the specific gravity of blood?

Chapter 4
Estimation of Hemoglobin

PROCEDURE STATION

Demonstrate the procedure of estimation of hemoglobin by Sahli's method up to the formation of acid hematin.

Checklist

1. Selects N/10 HCl
2. Puts the acid up to the 2 gm % mark in the hemoglobin tube
3. Selects the hemoglobin pipette
4. Takes blood up to the 20 mark in the pipette
5. Places the tube in the lower part of the tube and transfer the blood
6. Stirs the content.

QUESTION STATION

1. A man has a Hb of 16 gm%, find out
   a. The oxygen carrying capacity of his blood
   b. The iron content of his blood.
2. Name two other methods of estimating the hemoglobin?
3. Name three other types of hemoglobin?
4. Name the end product whose colour is matched with the standard?
5. The hemoglobin of a subject was estimated by Sahli's method.
   a. Which is the acid generally, used in this method?
   b. Can any other acid be used? Explain your answer?
   c. Explain the principle of the Sahli's method?
6. The hemoglobin of a subject was found to be 20 gm%
   a. Enumerate two physiological causes of the increase?
   b. Identify the experimental errors that could have resulted in an abnormal high/low reading?
   c. Calculate the oxygen carrying capacity of the subject's blood?
7. The given diagram/ tube shows the estimated value of Hb by the Sahli's method.

a. What is the value of Hb in gm%?
   b. Name one other method of estimation of hemoglobin?
   c. What is the normal range of Hb of an adult male and an infant?
8. The investigation was done to diagnose a patient of anemia.
   a. What is it called?
   b. What changes do you expect in a patient of anemia?
9. The hemoglobin of a pregnant woman was found to be 5 gm%
   a. What other information do you require to classify the type of anemia?
   b. What is the microscopic picture of iron deficiency anemia?

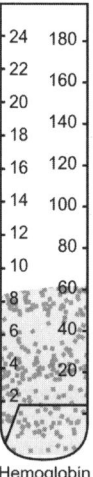

Chapter 5

Estimation of Red Blood Cell (RBC) Count

PROCEDURE STATION-1

Demonstrate the procedure of charging the chamber for doing RBC/ WBC count. Pipette filled with blood is provided.

Checklist

1. Cleans the chamber.
2. Cleans the cover slip.
3. Discards a few drops of solution.
4. Wipes the tip of pipette.
5. Places the pipette at 45° angle at the edge of cover slip.
6. Charges the chamber.
7. Chambers is adequately charged.
8. If inappropriately charged tries again after cleaning the previous one.
9. It is now adequately charged.

PROCEDURE STATION-2

Demonstrate the procedure of filling the pipette for doing RBC/ WBC count.

Checklist

1. Chooses the right pipette.
2. Chooses the right stain.
3. Fills blood upto the 0.5 mark.
4. Wipes the end of the pipette.
5. Fills the dilution fluid/stain up to 101/11 mark.
6. Mixes the content by rolling the pipette.

QUESTION STATION

1. The peripheral blood smear is placed in front of you.
   a. Comment on the RBCs.

Estimation of Red Blood Cell (RBC) Count

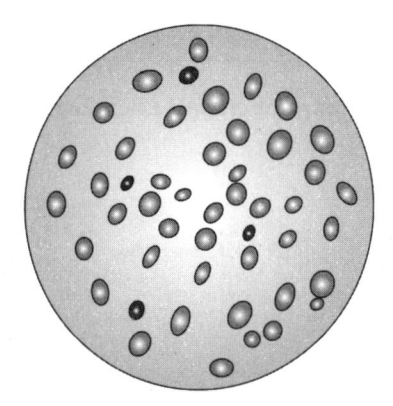

Peripheral smear showing anemia

    b. What is the normal size of the RBCs?
    c. How would you diagnose anemia on the basis of the peripheral smear?
2. Calculate the RBC count if number of cells counted is 400 (using Neubauer's chamber).
3. How do you calculate the dilution factor for RBC count?
4. The pictorial depiction of a Neubauer's chamber is given to you. Calculate the RBC count. Is it within normal limit? (Picture of Neubauer's chamber with RBC to be provided)
5. What is the practical importance of doing the RBC count?
6. Name the method used currently in clinics for doing the RBC count.
7. A 25-year-old lady comes to you with weakness. Name two investigations you would like to do?
8. A 35-year-old lady was treated with anemia due to iron deficiency.
    a. What was her blood picture before treatment likely to be?
    b. If the treatment was on the right lines, what is the blood picture likely to be now?
9. What factors help you to identify the RBC pipette?
10. Can the WBC pipette be used to calculate the RBC count? Explain.
11. The investigation was done during a routine hematological examination of a subject who is probably suffering from anemia.
    a. What is the investigation that has been carried out?
    b. What changes do you expect in a patient of anemia?
    c. Name the anticoagulant routinely used in this experiment and also mention its functional importance.
12. What other value is obtained by using the RBC count as one of its parameter?

13. This is a pipette routinely used for hemtological experiments.
    a. Identify the use.
    b. Mention one important characteristic feature.

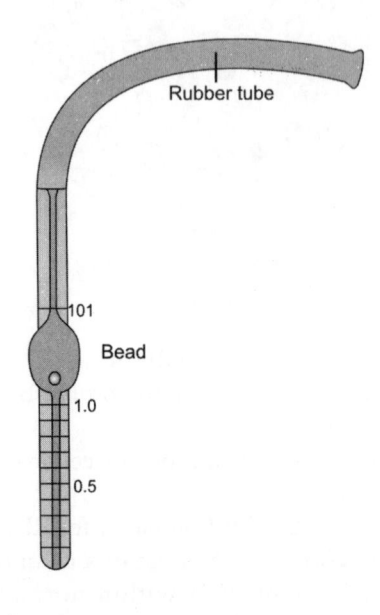

Chapter 6

Estimation of RBC Indices

1. The Hb value of a young adult was found to be 15 gm%, PCV 45% and RBC count 5 million/cubic mm.
   a. Calculate the MCV?
   b. What other information can you obtain from the above values?
   c. What is the importance of calculating the RBC indices?
2. Blood indices can be calculated using certain hematological investigations
   a. What do you understand by MCHC?
   b. What are the hematological investigations that must be done to? Calculate MCHC?
   c. What is the blood picture of a patient suspected of having microcytic hypochromic anemia?

Chapter 7

Determining of Osmotic Fragility of the RBC

QUESTION STATION

1. Shown below are test tubes with different percentages of saline. A drop of blood is added to each tube.

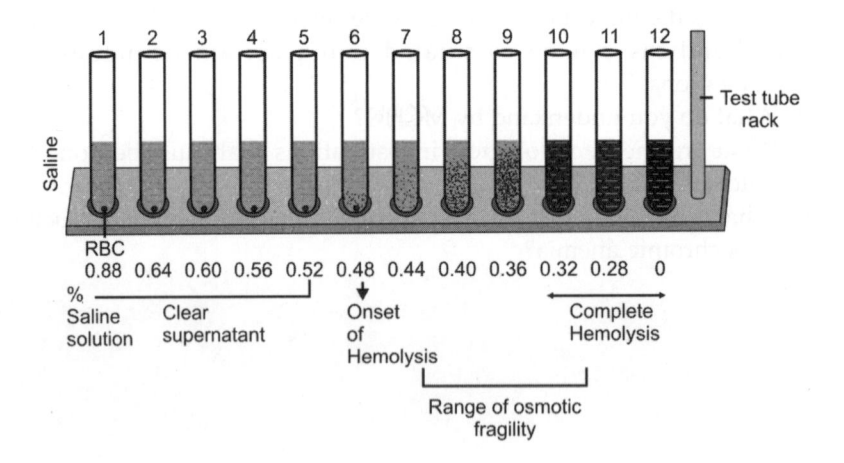

a. At what point is the onset of fragility?
b. At what point is fragility complete?
c. If the solution was vigorously shaken, what is the factor that can complicate results?
2. A patient has lot of fluid loss due to diarrhea and has to be given intravenous fluids. Four options namely, 5% glucose, 10% glucose, 15% glucose 0.6% saline are available. Which of the fluids you would like to transfuse and why?
3. Name two isotonic agents?
4. Name two conditions in which hemolysis occur *in vivo* in man?
5. The osmotic fragility of a cell was found to be 0.44.
   a. Comment on the above value?
   b. What happens to the osmotic fragility in G_6 PD deficiency?

c. Name two anticoagulants routinely used during hematology practical?
6. The osmotic fragility of a cell was found to be 0.30.
   a. Comment on the result with reasons?
   b. Name two conditions which could lead to hemolysis in the body?
7. The osmotic fragility was determined by the standard method.
   a. What is the normal range of osmotic fragility?
   b. Name one condition in which the osmotic fragility is:
      i. Increased
      ii. Decreased
   c. What is the solution that is routinely put inside the test-tubes?
   d. What is the principle of the method routinely used?
8. The diagram shows the method of determining the osmotic fragility of blood
   a. What is the solution that is put inside the test tubes?
   b. What is the normal range of osmotic fragility?
   c. What is the principle of the method routinely used?

Chapter 8

Determining of Erythrocyte Sedimentation Rate (ESR) and Packed Cell Volume (PCV)

QUESTION STATION

1. Two tubes A and B are shown to you.

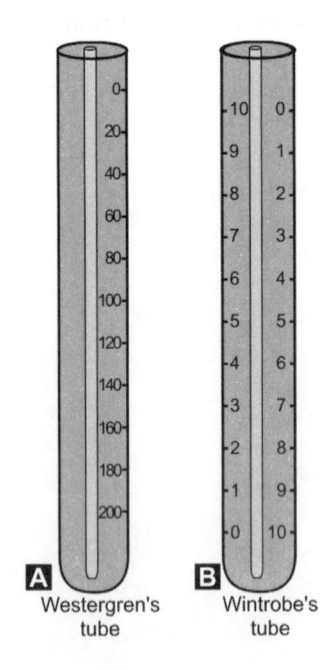

   A — Westergren's tube
   B — Wintrobe's tube

   a. Name them?
   b. What are they used for?
   c. Which of them is preferred and why?
2. A tube containing blood is centrifuged.
   a. Name the tube?
   b. What value is recorded by the above procedure?
   c. What other use can the above tube be put to in hematology experiments?

Determining of ESR and PCV

3. The ESR of a male patient was 5 mm in the first hour.
   a. Is the value normal?
   b. Name two indications of doing ESR.
   c. What is the physiological principle of ESR?
4. The packed cell volume of a subject was estimated by using standard procedure.

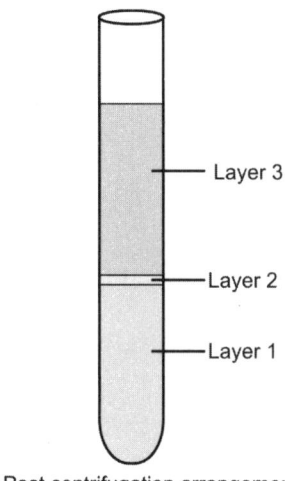

Post centrifugation arrangement of layers of blood

   a. What are the different layers seen?
   b. What change do you expect in a patient suffering from leukemia?
   c. What factors can affect the PCV?
5. The packed cell volume of a subject was estimated by using standard procedure.
   a. What is the normal range of PCV in an adult male?
   b. What is the clinical significance of doing the PCV count?
   c. What will happen to the PCV at high altitude? Explain your answer.
6. The ESR of a subject was 72 mm in the first hour.
   a. Interpret the result?
   b. Name two causes that could have resulted in the above picture?
   c. Write down the principle of the Westergren's method?
7. The ESR of an individual was estimated in the laboratory
   a. Identify the tube placed in front of you?
   b. Name the other method of estimating the ESR?
   c. Mention two factors that can affect the ESR?
8. The ESR of an individual was estimated in the laboratory
   a. What is the value?
   b. Why is it important to know if ESR has been measured in the first or the second hour?
   c. What is the normal value in an adult female?

9. The ESR of an individual was estimated in the laboratory by the Westergren's method
   a. What is the result?
   b. Name the other method. Which is preferred and why?
   c. What is the principle of ESR estimation?

Chapter 9

Estimation of Blood Groups

PROCEDURE STATION

Demonstrate the procedure for determining the blood group from the sample provided by the slide method.

Checklist

1. Selects a clean slide.
2. Selects anti A, anti B and anti Rh factor.
3. Selects normal saline for the control.
4. Marks the slide.
5. Puts anti A, anti B and anti Rh and saline in appropriate places.
6. Puts one drop of suspension for each.
7. Mixs the contents and wait for agglutination.
8. Reports correctly (by observing under the microscope).

QUESTION STATION

1. The slide shows agglutination with antiserum.

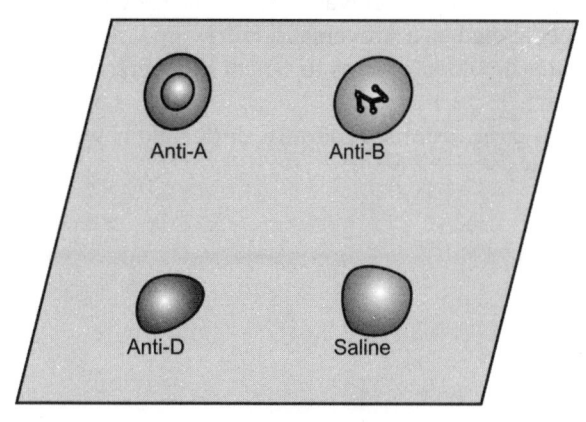

Red cell suspension added to antisera

a. Comment on the blood group?
b. Name the blood groups of patients to whom this patient can donate blood?
c. Name the blood groups of patients from whom this patient can receive blood?

2. The slide shows agglutination with anti A serum (slide to be provided).
   a. Comment on the blood group?
   b. What is the antigen present in the blood?
   c. What antibodies are likely to be present in the serum of this patient?

3. A person whose blood group is AB+ is about to receive transfusion.

   Donor 1. A   Donor 3. AB
   Donor 2. B   Donor 4. O

   a. From the donor's provided which can be selected and why?
   b. Name the precautions that need to be taken during a blood transfusion?

4. The blood group of a pregnant female is AB Rh +
   a. What could be the complications if the fetus is:
      i. Rh +ve
      ii. Rh –ve
   b. What precautions must be taken in subsequent pregnancies?

5. The blood group of a Rh –ve person was transfused to a Rh+ve recipient
   a. What do you expect will happen?
   b. Name the blood group that is called the 'universal donor'?
   c. Name the law that deals with blood groups?
   d. Name the antibodies that you expect to find in the blood group A+ve?

6. The blood group of a person was B+ve.
   a. Which antibodies do you expect in the serum?
   b. What is the class of antibodies generally present in the serum?
   c. Which types of antibodies are transferred via the placenta to the fetus?

7. The blood group of a person was found to be O+ve.
   a. Can he be labeled as a universal donor?
   b. Enumerate the blood groups to which this person can safely donate blood?
   c. Name two precautions generally undertaken while doing blood transfusion?

Chapter 10

Determination of Reticulocyte Count

QUESTION STATION

1. a. Identify the cell focused under the microscope.

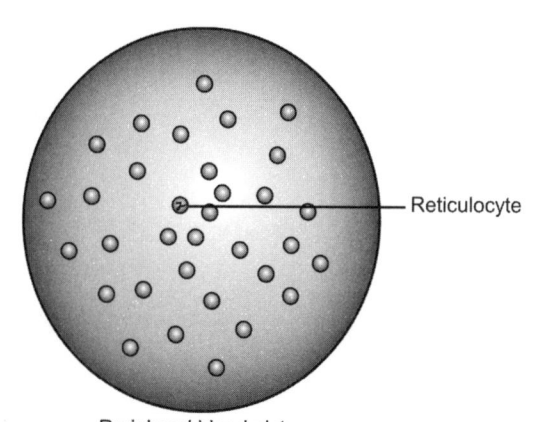

   Peripheral blood picture

   b. Name the stain that has been used?
   c. What is the percentage of the cells found in the normal adult male?
2. a. What do you understand by the term vital staining?
   b. In what conditions is vital staining done?
   c. What are the precautions taken while doing this staining?
3. A patient was being treated for iron deficiency anemia.
   a. Name two investigations that can be done to see if the treatment was successful?
   b. Which response is likely to precede the other as shown by the above investigations?
4. The reticulocyte count differs from other investigations routinely done in a hematology lab.
   a. Explain the above statement?

b. Give the normal value of reticulocyte count in:
   i. An adult
   ii. An infant.
c. What is the clinical importance of determining the reticulocyte count?
5. The picture of a cell focused under the oil immersion lens of a microscope is shown.
   a. Identify the cell?
   b. Enumerate the features that helped you to identify the cell?
   c. What is the staining that has been performed?

Chapter 11

Estimation of Total Leukocyte Count

PROCEDURE STATION-1

Demonstrate the procedure of filling the pipette in total leukocyte count.

Checklist
1. Chooses the right pipette.
2. Chooses the right stain.
3. Fills blood upto the 0.5 mark.
4. Wipes the end of the pipette.
5. Fills the dilution fluid/stain up to 11 mark.
6. Mixes the content by rolling the pipette.

PROCEDURE STATION-2

Demonstrate the procedure of charging the chamber in total leukocyte count.

Checklist
1. Cleans the chamber.
2. Cleans the cover slip.
3. Discards a few drops of solution.
4. Wipes the tip of pipette.
5. Places the pipette at 45° angle at the edge of cover slip.
6. Charges the chamber.
7. Chambers is adequately charged.
8. If inappropriately charged tries again after cleaning the previous one.
9. It is now adequately charged.

PROCEDURE STATION-3

Focus a chamber where counting of leukocytes is done.

Checklist
1. Selects an improved Neubauer's chamber.
2. Cleans it with appropriate material.
3. Places it on the microscope.

Objective Structured Practical Examination in Physiology

4. Adjusts the stage, mirror and the eyepiece.
5. Focuses the chamber in low power.

QUESTION STATION

The picture below shows cells as observed under the microscope.

2	4	2	1		1	4	9	2
4	5	2	0		4	2	6	3
9	7	6	4		2	0	4	8
10	9	7	5		1	4	2	4

2	4	4	3		1	1	3	4
3	2	4	9		1	2	8	4
4	4	5	7		2	7	8	2
5	9	2	6		9	7	6	2

1. Calculate the total leukocyte count?
2. Derive the dilution factor and the multiplication factor for the total leukocyte count?
3. A patient had high grade fever.
    a. Name the hematological investigations that would help you to investigate the cause of fever in this patient?
4. The TLC of a patient was 16000. On treatment with antibiotics the patient responded. What change do you expect in the TLC?
5. Name the fluid used to do the TLC. Can RBCs be visualized in the preparation? Explain your answer?
6. The diagram depicts an improved Neubauer's chamber used for estimating the TLC.
    a. Calculate the TLC?

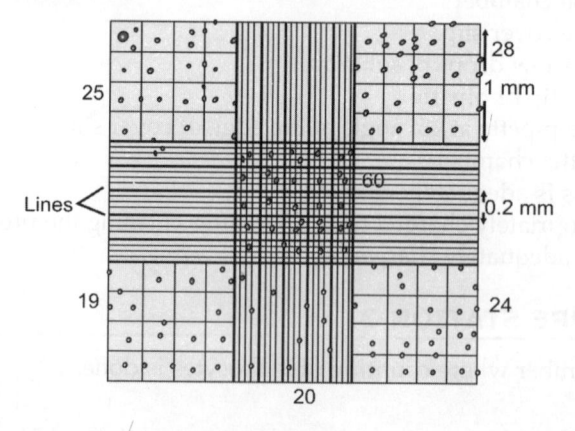

b. Explain the basis of the dilution and multiplication factor?
c. Mention two important precautions mandatory while doing the TLC?

Chapter 12
Preparation of a Smear and Differential Leukocyte Count

PROCEDURE STATION-1

Demonstrate the procedure of making a smear using the sample of blood provided.

Checklist

1. Selects a good slide.
2. Cleans the slide.
3. Selects a good spreader slide.
4. Takes blood in a dropper.
5. Puts an appropriate amount of blood on the slide.
6. Holds the spreader at 45° angle.
7. Movement are smooth.
8. A good smear is made.

PROCEDURE STATION-2

Demonstrate the procedure of staining the smear provided for differential leukocyte count (disregard time period for staining).

Checklist

1. Arranges the smears for staining.
2. Covers the smear with Leishman stain.
3. Covers the smear with distilled water.
4. Washes out the stain.
5. Keeps it for drying.

QUESTION STATION

1. The DLC shows N40 L45 E10 M5 B0
   a. Comment on the report?
2. The DLC shows N70 L25 E1 M4 B0
   a. Comment on the report?
3. The DLC shows N70 L20 E7 M3 B0
   a. Comment on the report?

Objective Structured Practical Examination in Physiology

4. The smear shows a slide stained for DLC.
   a. Identify one probable error done during staining?
   b. How is it likely to affect the result?

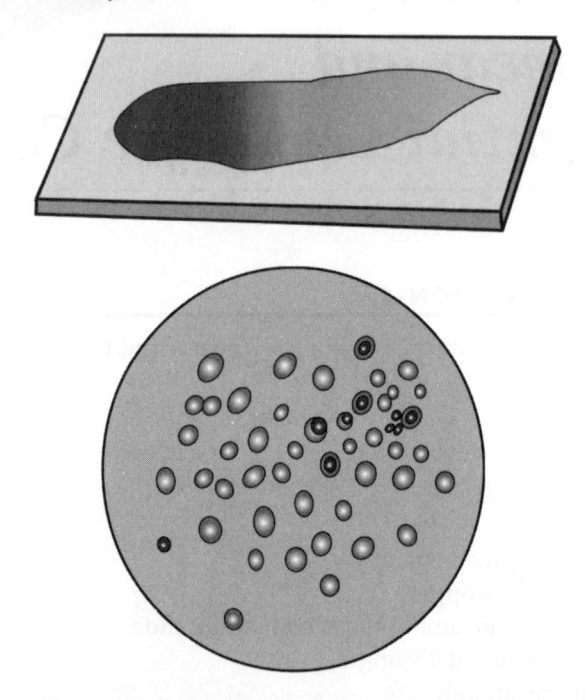

5. Two smears are provided to you.
   a. Identify the ideal smear?
   b. Name two errors seen in the other smear?
6. Enumerate 5 points of information that a peripheral smear can provide?
7. Why is buffered water used to prepare the stain?
8. Name two stains that can be used to stain a DLC?
9. The given smear has been stained using Leishman's stain
       a. Why is it important to fix the smear before staining?

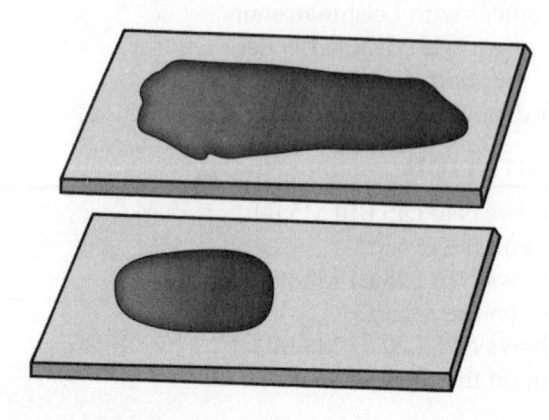

Preparation of a Smear and Differential Leukocyte Count

    b. What component of the stain acts as a fixative?
    c. Why must the stain be acetone free?
10. The given smear has been stained using Leishman's stain
    a. What is the importance of using buffered water during staining?
    b. Describe the appearance of eosinophil granules?
    c. What in your opinion is the clinical value of a peripheral smear?
11. The DLC report of a child was follows—N32 L55 E10 M2 B1
    a. Comment on the report?
    b. Mention two clinical conditions that could result in the above blood picture?
12. A smear is focused under the microscope
    a. Identify the cell focused?
    b. Mention two of its identifying features?
    c. Name one condition in which the count of the cell focused above is
        i. Increased
        ii. Decreased.
    d. What staining has been done?
    e. What are the constituents of the cell that help it to perform its function?
13. Samples of different smears made are kept in front of you
    a. Identify the ideal/good smear?
    b. Mention some of the lacunae observed in the other smears?
    c. What is the standard time period for Leishman's staining?

Chapter 13
Determining of Absolute Eosinophil Count

PROCEDURE STATION

Demonstrate the procedure of estimating the absolute eosinophil count after filling the pipette and before charging the chamber. Disregard the time period rules.

Checklist

1. Checks the value of fluid in the pipette.
2. Gently shake the pipette in the palm.
3. Takes a petridish.
4. Moisten a filter paper.
5. Puts the filter paper on the petridish.
6. Keeps a filled pipette on it.
7. Another moistened filter paper is taken.
8. This filter paper is placed under the cover of the petridish.
9. The pipette is removed.
10. A few drops are discarded.

QUESTION STATION

1. The diagram shows a charged chamber for absolute eosinophil count.
    a. Calculate the value of absolute eosinophil count?
    b. Mention another method which may be an indirect method of estimating the absolute eosinophil count?
    c. Name the stain used for this experiment?
2. The cell focused under a microscope is shown.
    a. Identify the cell?
    b. Give its two characteristic features?
    c. What are the unique constituents of the cell that helped it to perform it's functions?
3. The picture of Neubauer's chamber is shown below. The chamber is charged for eosinophil count.
    a. In which squares do you count eosinophils?

Determining of Absolute Eosinophil Count

   b. Calculate the eosinophil count?
   c. Name one condition in which the eosinophil count increases?
4. The picture of Neubauer's chamber is shown below. The chamber is charged for eosinophil count.
   a. What is the multiplication factor derived for this experiment?
   b. Name the diluting fluid used for eosinophil count?
   c. What is the principle used for the staining?
5. The picture of a cell focused under 100X is shown
   a. Identify the cell focused?
   b. What are the characteristic features of this cell?
   c. Name one condition in which the cell count
      i. Increases
      ii. Decreases.
6. A 4-year-old boy has worm infestation and is also having some allergic symptoms. A routine blood examination including the DLC was done.
   a. What changes do you expect in the DLC?
   b. Name one additional investigation you would like to do in this case?
   c. What is the reason for the changes in the cell count?
7. The diagram shows a charged Neubauer's chamber during the estimation of eosinophil count
   a. What is the eosinophil count?
   b. Name two conditions in which the eosinophil count increases?
   c. What types of granules are present in the eosinophil?
8. The diagram shows a charged Neubauer's chamber during the estimation of eosinophil count.

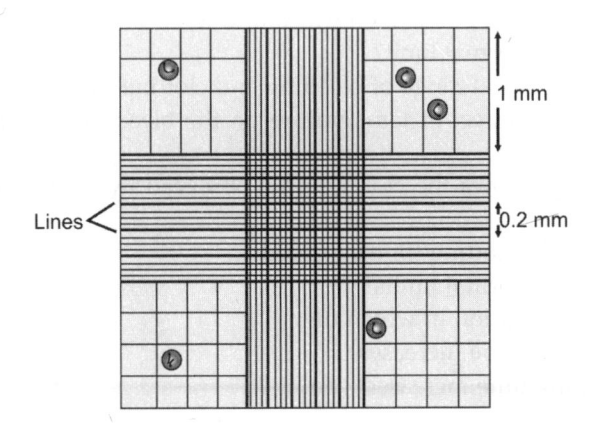

   a. What is the eosinophil count?
   b. What is the name of the stain used for the eosinophil count?
   c. What do you understand by the term "absolute " and "relative" eosinophil count?

Chapter 14

Determination of Bleeding and Clotting Time

QUESTION STATION

1. The clotting time of a person was found to be 5 minutes.
   a. Is it within the normal range?
   b. What is the applied importance of estimating clotting time?
   c. Explain why thrombocytopenia decreases the bleeding time but not the clotting time?
2. The clotting time of a person was 4 minutes.
   a. Enumerate the methods of determining the clotting time?
   b. Enumerate the factors that can effect the clotting time?
   c. Define prothrombin time. What is its normal value? Interpret the results?
   d. Enumerate two precautions undertaken while performing:
      i. Clotting time
      ii. Bleeding time.
3. The bleeding time of a person was found to be 3 minutes
   a. Is it within normal limit?
   b. Give the normal range of bleeding and clotting time?
   c. What is the effect of temperature on the bleeding and the clotting time?
4. The diagram shows the clotting time observed by using the capillary method.
   a. What is the clotting time observed?
   b. Is it within normal limits?
   c. Name a condition in which the:
      i. Bleeding time increases
      ii. Clotting time increases.

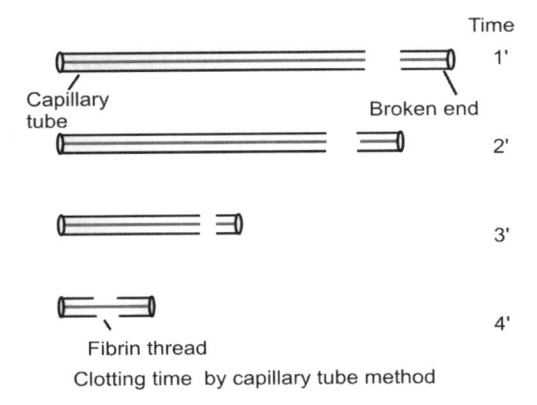

Determination of Bleeding and Clotting Time

Clotting time by capillary tube method

(Capillary tube, Broken end, Fibrin thread — Time: 1', 2', 3', 4')

5. The bleeding time of an individual is shown on the filter paper
   a. What is the bleeding time observed?
   b. Is it within normal limit?
   c. Mention another method of estimating the bleeding time?

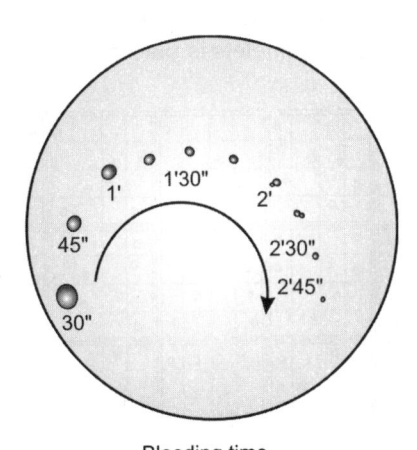

Bleeding time

(Markings: 30", 45", 1', 1'30", 2', 2'30", 2'45")

Chapter 15

Determination of Platelet Count

QUESTION STATION

1. A few bottles containing different fluids used in hematology estimations are provided to you.
   a. Identify the fluid used for platelet count?
   b. Write and draw how the platelets look like under the microscope?
   c. Give the normal range of platelet count?
2. A chamber charged with platelets is placed in front of you.

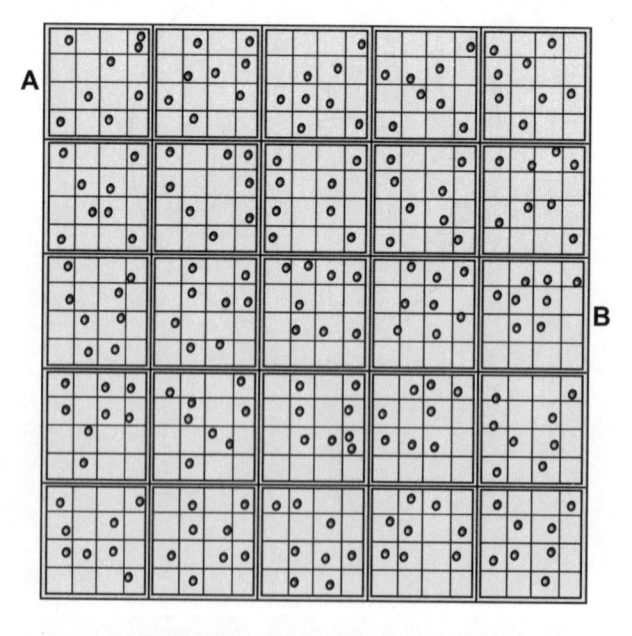

   a. Count the number of platelets in A and B?
   b. If the number in the count of A and B is drastically different what information does it give to you?
   c. What is the multiplication factor in the calculation of the platelet count?

3. The platelet count of an individual is found to be 2 - 5 lac/mm
   a. What can be the expected bleeding time?
   b. What is the effect of splenectomy on the clotting and bleeding time?
   c. Enumerate two functions of platelets.
4. A 20-year-old female presented with petechial hemorrhages.
   a. What investigation would you like to do?
   b. Name the factor whose deficiency is responsible for hemophilia?
   c. Describe how you would test the integrity of platelets?

Chapter 16

Study of Bone Marrow

1. Identify the cell?
2. To which series of cells does it belong?
3. Name the cell which occurs before and the cell which appears after it in the series?
4. Name one factor that can increase its production?
5. Name one factor that can decrease its production?
6. Is it found in normal peripheral smear?

Unit 2

Amphibian Experiments

17. Experimental Set-up and Simple Muscle Twitch
18. Effect of Temperature on the Simple Muscle Twitch
19. Effect of Two Successive Stimuli on Skeletal Muscle Contraction
20. Effect of Increasing Strength of Stimulus on Skeletal Muscle Contraction
21. Effect of Increasing Frequency of Stimulus on Skeletal Muscle Contraction
22. After Loaded and Free Loaded Condition
23. Genesis of Fatigue in Skeletal Muscle
24. Recording of Isometric Contraction
25. Determination of Conduction Velocity of the Sciatic Nerve
26. Recording of Normal Cardiogram and Effect of Temperature on Normal Cardiogram
27. Properties of the Cardiac Muscle
28. Effect of Stimulation of the Vagus Nerve and White Crescentic Line on the Cardiogram
29. Effect of Some Variables on the Isolated Frog's Heart and the Intact Frog's Heart

Chapter 17

Experimental Set-up and Simple Muscle Twitch

The graph below shows a simple muscle twitch recorded.

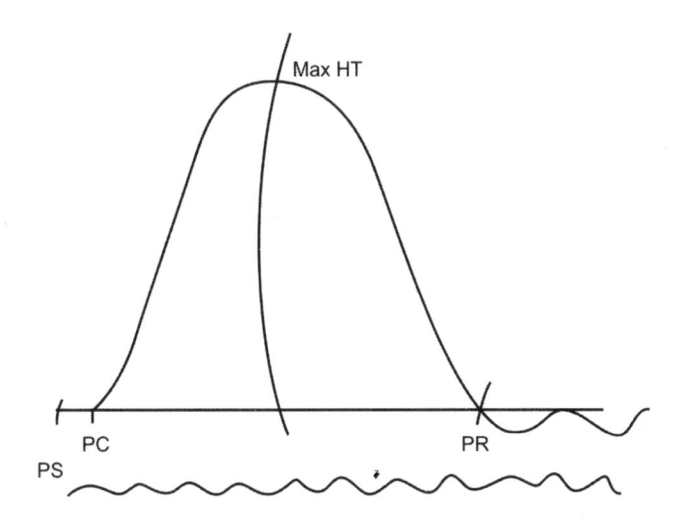

1. Calculate the latent period?
2. Name and state how two factors can influence the latent period?
3. Calculate the contraction and relaxation period. Give the significance of each?
4. What is the time duration of the contraction if the frequency of the tuning fork is 100Hz?
5. What is the importance of keeping the drum in circuit?
6. Is the contraction recorded isotonic or isometric?
7. Draw where you would expect to record the action potential in this diagram?
8. Calculate the tetanizing frequency of the muscle from this graph?
9. If the load suspended from the lever is increased what changes do you expect in the graph?
10. What is the name given to the nerve and the muscle?

11. What is the effect of increasing the strength of stimulus on the SMT?
12. How can the strength of the stimulus be changed?
13. What is the importance of measuring the height of contraction?
14. Which period (contraction or relaxation) do you expect to be longer and why?
15. What is the composition of amphibian ringer solution?
16. Name two reasons for using frog to demonstrate physiology experiments?
17. What type of stimulus is given, i.e. subthreshold, threshold or suprathreshold in a SMT?
18. What are the ionic changes taking place during the action potential?
19. What are the ionic changes taking place during the contraction and the relaxation period?
20. Point out the error in the circuit?

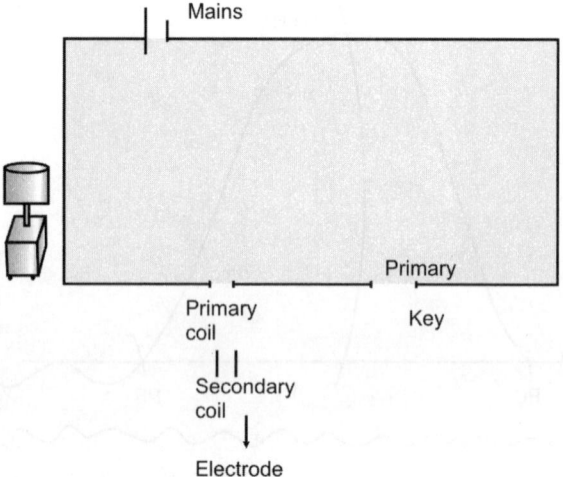

Error: Kymograph not included in circuit

Chapter 18
Effect of Temperature on the Simple Muscle Twitch

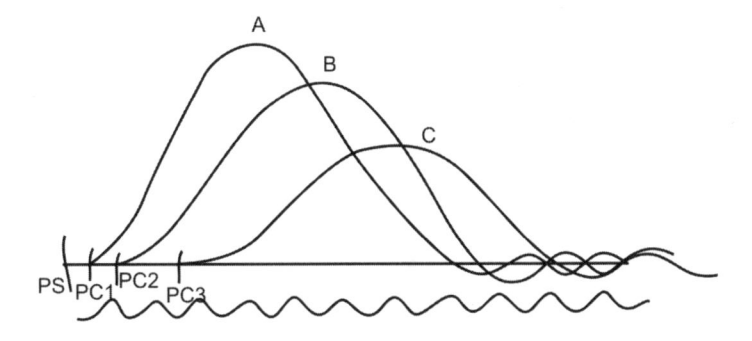

The above graph of the recording of hot and cold ringer is presented in front of you.
(*Graph similar to SMT but three graphs will be overlapping, with different latent period and height of contraction*)

1. What is the effect of adding hot and cold ringer on the simple muscle twitch?
2. Calculate the latent period of the normal and "hot ringer" recording.
3. What is the maximum temperature to which you can heat the ringer? What will happen beyond and why?
4. What is the effect of decrease in temperature on the contraction period and the height of contraction?
5. What is the importance of effect of increased and decreased temperature on the skeletal muscle contraction?
6. What happens to the duration of various phases SMT if the temperature is decreased to 4°C?
7. What happens to the duration of various phases SMT if the temperature is increased to 45°C?

Chapter 19

Effect of Two Successive Stimuli on Skeletal Muscle Contraction

1. The below graph showing effect of two successive stimuli on skeletal muscle contraction is given to you.
   a. Identify graph (A, B, C, D), in which the stimulus is given in the later half of the latent period?

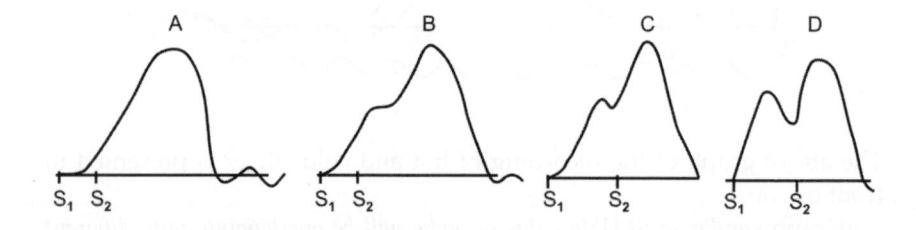

   b. What type of stimulus is used (maximal/submaximal/supramaximal) and why?
   c. If only one graph is recorded, where have you probably given the second stimulus?
   d. Why is the height of contraction more when you give the second stimulus in the early relaxation period?
2. The circuit used in the experiment effect of two successive stimuli on skeletal muscle contraction is made in front of you.

Effect of Two Successive Stimuli on Skeletal Muscle Contraction

a. Point out the error in the circuit?

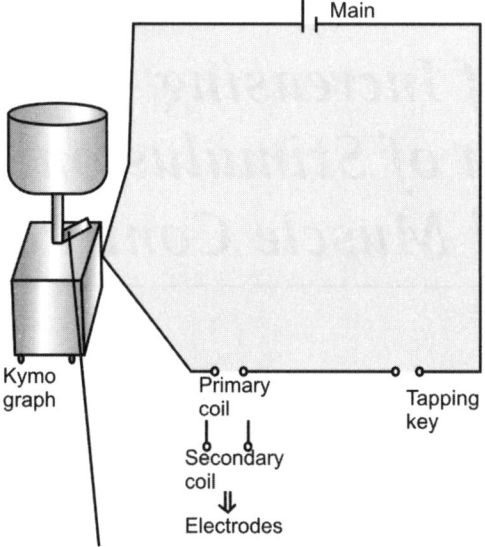

Error prongs not seperated to give two successive stimuli

(Diagram labels: Main, Kymo graph, Primary coil, Secondary coil, Electrodes, Tapping key)

b. Draw the expected graph if you give the second stimulus in the contraction period of the first stimulus?

3. Draw a diagram to show the pattern of the SMT recorded when the second stimulus is given:
   a. During the early latent period of the twitch.
   b. During the contraction period of the twitch.
   c. What do you understand by the term "beneficial" effect?
4. The effect of two successive stimuli was demonstrated
   a. What is the special feature of the experimental set up of this demonstration?
   b. Is the drum included in the circuit?
   c. Draw a diagram to explain the effect of giving the second stimulus in the late latent period of the first stimulus?
5. Identify the error in the circuit?

Chapter 20

Effect of Increasing Strength of Stimulus on Skeletal Muscle Contraction

On the X-axis is the distance in cm between the primary and the secondary coil. On the Y-axis is the height of contraction (in cm) record.

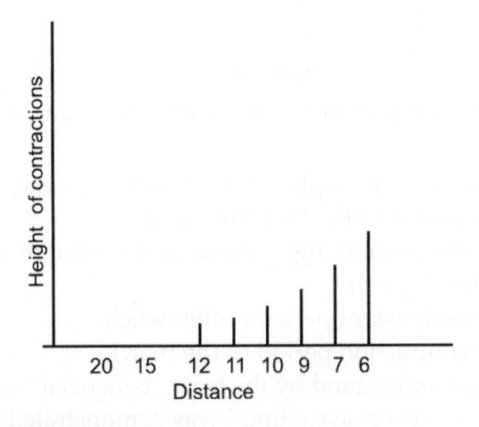

[Graph: Height of contractions vs Distance, with x-axis values 20 15 12 11 10 9 7 6]

1. Explain how the strength of current is increased?
2. What is the type of current?
3. Explain how the height of contraction increases and then remains constant after some time?
4. Define subthreshold current?
5. What is a motor unit?
6. What is the difference between threshold and maximal stimulus and Why?
7. Does this preparation obey the all or none law?
8. What is the physiological importance of this practical in humans?

Chapter 21

Effect of Increasing Frequency of Stimulus on Skeletal Muscle Contraction

The graphical recording of stimulation of the frog's gastrocnemius muscle via the sciatic nerve is provided below Graph.

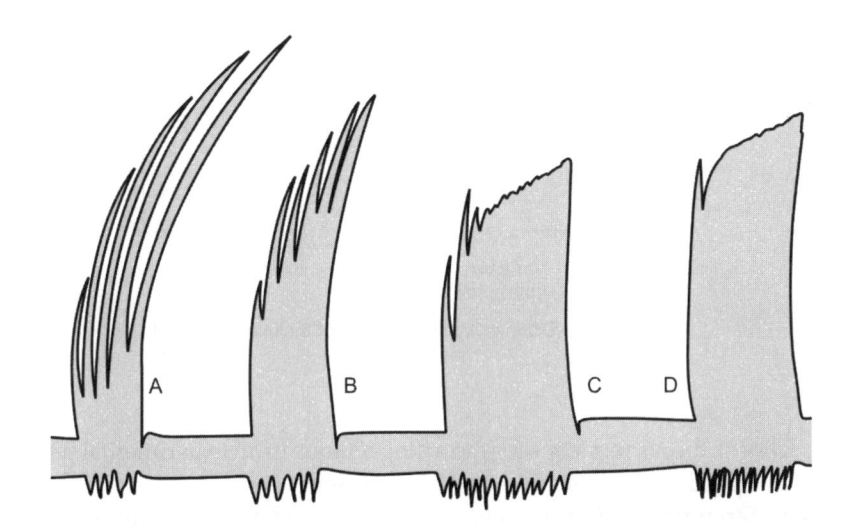

1. Identify A, B, C, and D.
2. What are the difference between A and B, B and C, C and D?
3. Name the instrument which is used to increase the frequency of stimulus.
4. Define twitch duration, tetanising frequency, summation, tetanus and tetany.
5. Can the cardiac muscle be tetanised? Give reasons for your answer.
6. Name two precautions that are to be taken in this experiment.
7. What is the comparison between the tension developed in this experiment and that during the simple muscle twitch?

8. What is the physiological relevance of this practical?
9. Do muscles in vivo get tetanized? Give reasons for your answer?
10. Differentiate between tetanus and contracture; tetanus and rigor.
11. Draw (a) Complete, and (b) Incomplete tetanus.
12. Explain what you understand by the term rigor mortis?
13. An error has been deliberately made in the circuit of the experiment to demonstrate the property of tetanus. Identify?

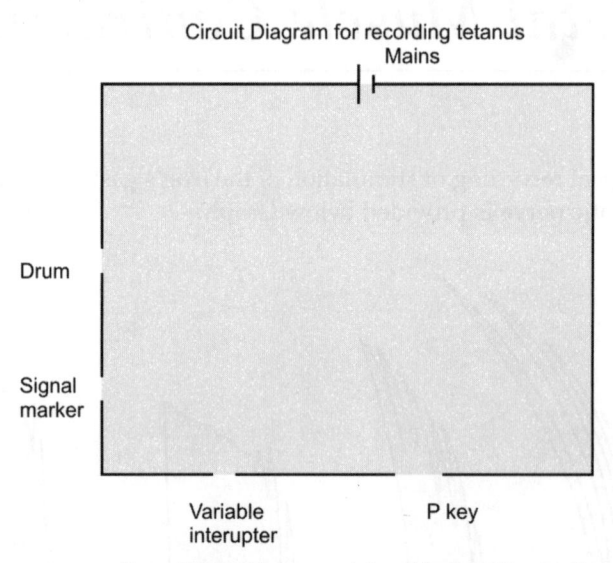

Circuit Diagram for recording tetanus
Mains

Drum

Signal marker

Variable interupter

P key

Error: Drum or kymograph is not included in circuit

14. Choose the correct steps for recording tetanus in an experimental setup.
    a. Speed of drum should be 12.5 mm/sec.
    b. Strength of stimulus is adjusted to get a maximal stimulus.
    c. Variable interrupter is included in the circuit.
    d. Drum is not to be included in the circuit.
    e. Include Kneef's hammer for delivering high frequency stimuli.
    f. Speed of drum should be 640 mm/sec.
    g. Include drum in the circuit.
    h. Open prongs of the strikes.
15. What do you understand by the terms?
    a. Staircase effect
    b. Treppe.

16. What is the difference between tetanus and fatigue?
17. What will happen if a calcium blocker is provided in the extracellular fluid?
18. What will happen is rest is given to the muscle in between repeated contraction?

Chapter 22

After Loaded and Free Loaded Condition

Diagrams (Below) show the effect of free and after loaded condition on the skeletal muscle contraction.

1. Identify the graphs for free loaded, afterloaded, moving and stationary drum (A, B, C, D)?

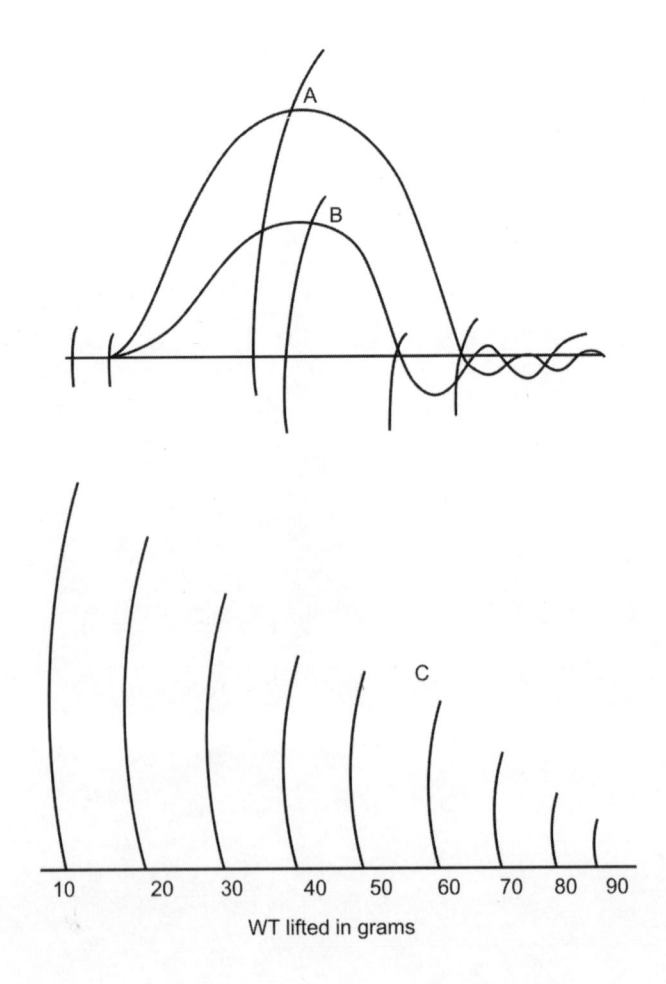

WT lifted in grams

After Loaded and Free Loaded Condition

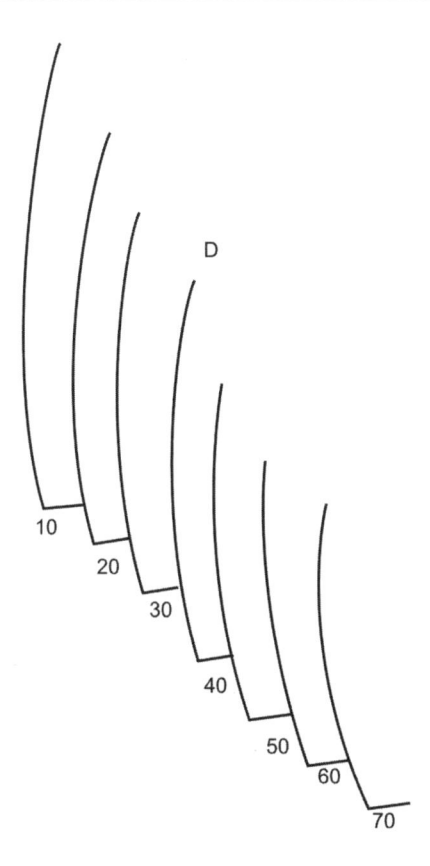

2. What do you understand by the term free and after loaded?
3. Give one example of a free and after loaded condition in the human body?
4. Calculate the work done in the free loaded condition given the weight as 20 gm and the height of contraction as 4 cm?
5. Explain diagrammatically the formula for calculating the height of contraction?
6. What do you understand by the term optimal load? What happens to the amount of work done or efficiency of the muscle when it is lifting optimal load?
7. What do you understand by the term resting or optimal length?
8. At what length can a muscle develop maximal active tension?
9. Can free and after loaded condition be applied to the cardiac muscle? Explain the clinical relevance?
10. Identify which is the free loaded and which is the afterloaded condition?
11. How do you calculate the work done in the after loaded condition?
12. Calculate the work done in the free loaded condition?

13. What difference do you expect in the work done in the free and afterloaded condition?
14. The work done in a free loaded condition was 2.04 Kgm. With subsequent increase in weight added, what change do you expect in the work done and why? Define the terms:
    a. Equilibrium length
    b. Resting length.
15. Work done was compared in a free loaded and after loaded condition. In which case more work is done and why? Give an example each of
    a. Free loaded condition
    b. After loaded condition.
16. Work done was compared in a free loaded and after loaded condition. What do you understand by the terms optimal length and optimal load? Explain how you experimentally create an after loaded condition?
17. The circuit of a practical conducted in the laboratory has been made. We have deliberately made an error in the circuit. Identify the error?

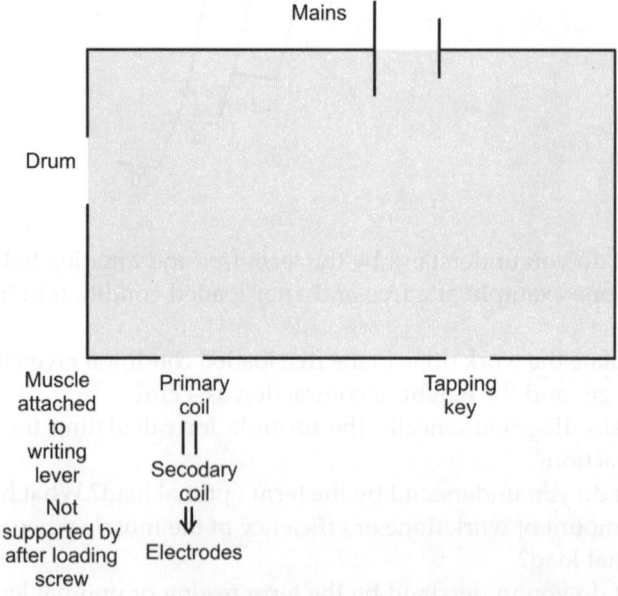

Mains

Drum

Muscle attached to writing lever
Not supported by after loading screw

Primary coil

Secodary coil ⇓

Tapping key

Electrodes

Error: After loading screw is not used for recording effect of after loaded condition

Chapter 23

Genesis of Fatigue in Skeletal Muscle

1. Define the term fatigue?
2. Explain why height of contraction first increases and then decreases.
3. What is the site of fatigue in an amphibian preparation? How will you confirm?
4. What is the site of human fatigue?
5. Give an example of human fatigue?
6. What is the cause of fatigue?
7. How does fatigue differ from tetanus?
8. How can muscles be prevented from undergoing fatigue during exercise?
9. Explain how a person exercising regularly will have a delayed onset of fatigue?
10. Study the given graph (Below) and explain the basis of contraction 1, 2, 3, 70 and direct stimulation of the muscle.

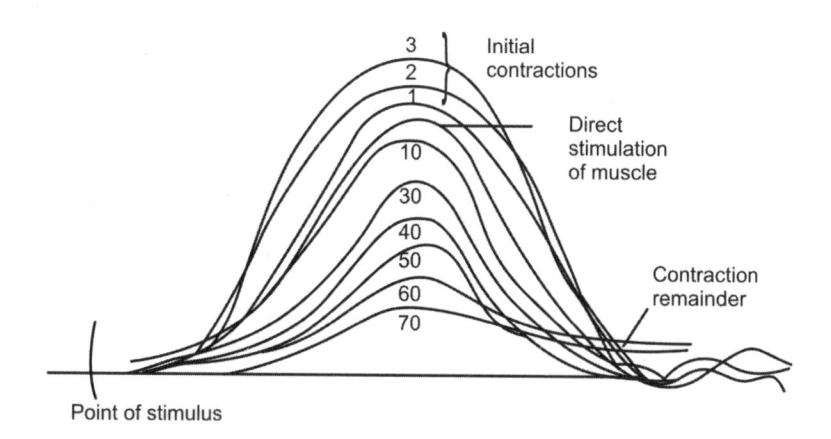

11. The graph shows the phenomenon of fatigue in a nerve muscle preparation on repeated stimulation.
    a. What is the site of fatigue? Is it the same in the case of a human muscle?
    b. Suggest an innovation/addition to demonstrate the site of fatigue?
12. The graph shows a "phenomenon" recorded on repeated stimulation of nerve-muscle preparation.
    a. What is the phenomenon called?
    b. Explain the physiological basis of this phenomenon?
13. In an experimental set up to record a simple muscle twitch, repeated stimuli were given.
    a. Why is the amplitude of the second contraction more than the first?
    b. How would you demonstrate that the muscle is not the site of fatigue?
    c. What in your opinion is the cause of fatigue?
14. In an experimental set up to demonstrate the phenomena of fatigue in a frog's gastrocnemius-sciatic nerve preparation
    a. Enumerate two causes that could have resulted in fatigue earlier?
    b. Can the phenomenon of fatigue be reversed? Explain your answer.

Chapter 24

Recording of Isometric Contraction

1. By definition what is the difference between isotonic and isometric contraction?
2. Name two differences in the setup between isotonic and isometric contraction?
3. In which case more external work is done and why?
4. Give an example each of isotonic and isometric contraction?
5. What do you understand by the term active and passive tension?

Chapter 25

Determination of Conduction Velocity of the Sciatic Nerve

The diagram (Below) shows the record obtained during the experimental recording of conduction velocity of the sciatic nerve preparation of the frog.

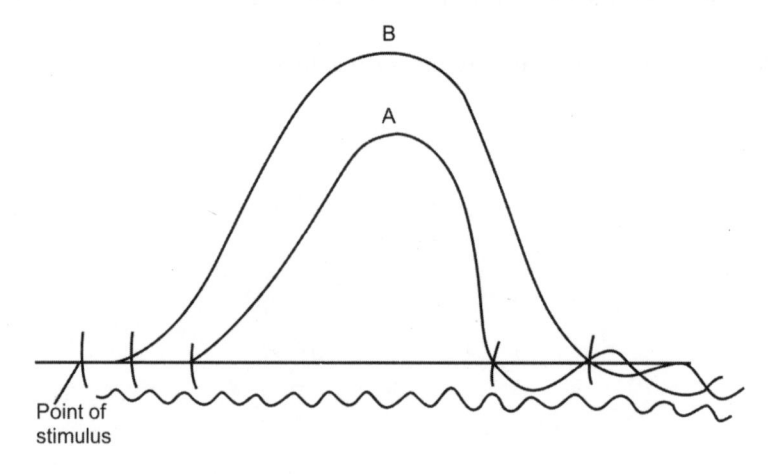

(Two SMT will be provided; the one of muscle end will have shorter latent period with same point of stimulus)
1. Identify A or B, which is the curve when the stimulus is given to the vertebral or the muscle end of the experimental preparation?
2. Which response will be higher and why?
3. Why are the latent periods different in the two cases?
4. Explain how the two curves are obtained experimentally?
5. Write the formula of calculating conduction velocity.
6. How is the graph used to calculate the conduction velocity of the nerve?
7. Name two muscles in the human body whose conduction velocity can be found out?
8. How is the length of the nerve fiber calculated?
9. What is the conduction velocity of A α, A α, and C fibers?
10. Name two causes of decreased nerve conduction velocity.

Determination of Conduction Velocity of the Sciatic Nerve

11. Can the conduction velocity be increased? Explain your answer.
12. The graph shows the SMT obtained when stimulating two ends of a sciatic nerve.
    a. Calculate the conduction velocity of the nerve from the graph?
    b. What are the factors that affect the conduction velocity?
13. The graph shows the two SMT recorded during the experiment of calculating the conduction velocity of sciatic nerve.
    a. Calculate the conduction velocity?
    b. How are the nerve fibers classified on the basis of their conduction velocity?
14. The graphs of conduction velocity of the frog's sciatic nerve are shown.
    a. Identify the graph of the vertebral end and the muscle end (A or B)?
    b. What is the relationship between the diameter and conduction velocity in:
        i. A myleinated nerve
        ii. Unmyleinated nerve.
15. In an experimental set up to record the conduction velocity of a frog's sciatic nerve:
    a. What important point has to be kept in mind while doing the experiment?
    b. How can you measure conduction velocity in a man?
    c. What is the clinical importance of measuring conduction velocity in a man?
16. Point out the errors in the circuit.

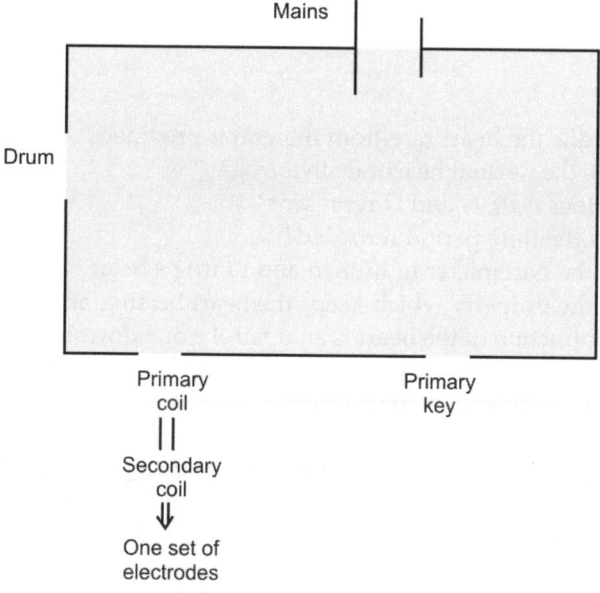

Error in circuit: Two sets of stimulating are necessary for conduction velocity

Chapter 26

Recording of Normal Cardiogram and Effect of Temperature on Normal Cardiogram

The graph (Below) of a normal cardiogram is shown in front of you.

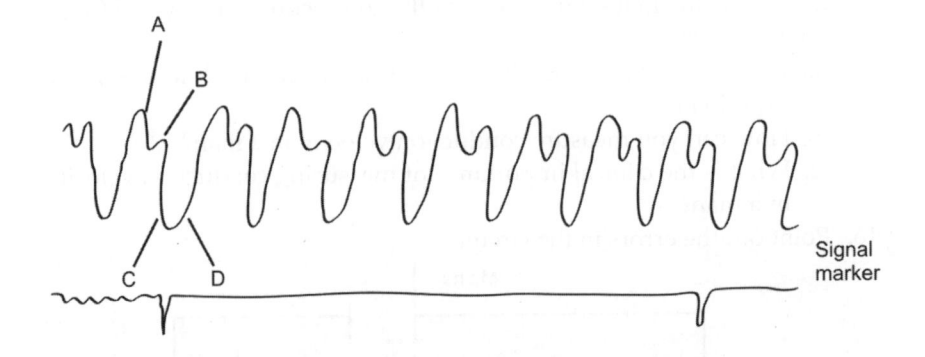

1. Determine the heart rate from the graph provided?
2. What is the normal heart rate in a frog?
3. What does A, B, C and D represent?
4. How is the time period recorded?
5. Name the pacemaker in human and in frog's heart?
6. Name the property which keeps the heart beating on its own?
7. The contraction of the heart is an upstroke or a downstroke and why?
8. What is the normal speed of drum in this experimental setup?
9. Trace the pathway of contraction?
10. Name two important precautions during this experiment?
11. What is the effect of adding warm and cold ringer on the heart?
12. What is the physiological importance of knowing the effect of temperature on the heart?

13. Can the findings of this experiment extrapolated to observations in the humans. Explain?
14. Why do we use the frog for this experiment?
15. What is the difference between an intact and an isolated heart preparation?
16. Name the different components of a cardiogram?
17. Point out the error in the circuit (any error can be made)?

Chapter 27

Properties of the Cardiac Muscle

1. Name two properties of the cardiac muscle that can be easily demonstrated?
2. What is a heart block and how is it produced?
3. Draw a diagram to show heart block?
4. Can heart block be produced in man? How?
5. What happens to the contractility of heart after a heart block?
6. Draw diagrams to show atleast two varieties of heart block in man?
7. Name the site of tying the first and the second stannous ligature?
8. What time does it take for the cardiac contractility to return after tying the first, the second stannous ligature?
9. What name is given to the contractility of the heart which returns after the second stannous ligature? What is the rate of contraction in this case?
10. What is the danger associated with heart block clinically?
11. Observe the diagrams given on the next page: State the property of the heart depicted in the diagram?
12. What do you understand by the term extrasystole and compensatory pause?
13. Explain whether extrasystole can occur clinically in man?
14. Explain diagrammatically what you understand by the term summation of subminimal stimuli?
15. What is the clinical importance of this property summation of subminimal stimuli?

Properties of the Cardiac Muscle

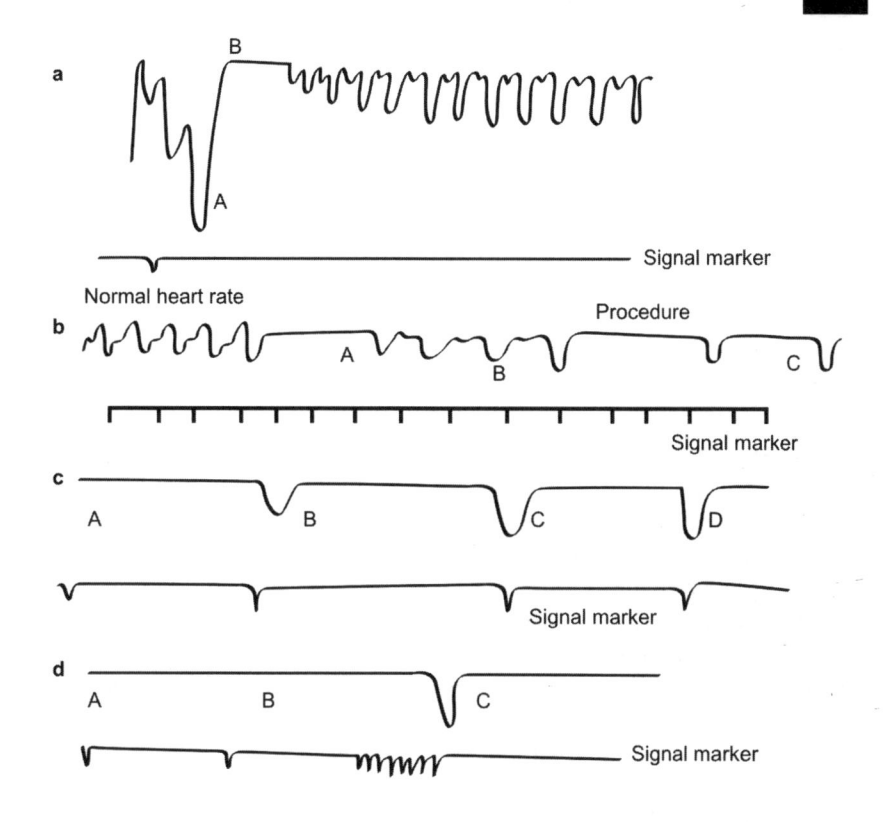

16. Study the Graph **a** and identify A and B?
17. Study the Graph **b** and identify A, B and C?
18. Identify the phenomenon occurring after studying the Graph **c**?
19. Identify the phenomenon occurring after studying the Graph **d**?
20. The frog's heart preparation is used to demonstrate the properties of the heart.
    a. What is the rhythm normally followed by the heart muscle?
    b. Does the cardiac muscle obey the all or none law? What is the property of the heart demonstrated by this?
21. Using a frog's heart preparation:
    a. Enumerate all the properties of the heart that can be demonstrated?
    b. Enumerate which experiments can be performed after the second stannius ligature is tied?
22. The experiment to demonstrate all or none law was performed using the frog's heart preparation:
    a. What result do you expect to get? Explain diagrammatically?
    b. What property of the cardiac muscle is depicted by the all or none law?
    c. Explain why the cardiac muscle cannot be tetanized?

23. Diagrammatically explain what you understand by the term:
    a. Beneficial effect
    b. All or none law.
24. An experiment to demonstrate the idioventicular rhythm was carried out:
    a. What is the rate of idioventricular rhythm?
    b. What precautions have to be taken during this experiment?
    c. How long does it take for the idioventricular rhythm to develop?
25. Choose the correct steps undertaken in the experiment for the all or none law.
    a. Tie the stannius ligature.
    b. Stimulate the heart with subthreshold stimuli.
    c. Stimulate the heart with threshold stimuli.
    d. Wait for 30 sec after each step.
    e. Wait for 5 sec after each step
    f. Stimulate the heart with threshold stimuli in quick succession.
    g. Speed of drum 12.5 mm/sec.
    h. Speed of drum 2.5 mm/sec.
    i. Stimulate the heart during early diastole.
26. Choose the correct steps undertaken in the experiment for recording an extrasystole:
    a. Speed of drum should be 12.5 mm/sec
    b. Simulate the beating heart with a single stimulus
    c. Simulate the quiescent heart with a threshold stimulus in quick
    d. Simulate the quiescent heart with a subthreshold stimulus
    e. Record a normal cardiogram
    f. Tie the stannius ligature.
27. A graph shown extrasystole and compensatory pause is shown to you, what is the normal duration of the event?

Chapter 28

Effect of Stimulation of the Vagus Nerve and White Crescentic Line on the Cardiogram

Study the graphs given below and answer the following questions.

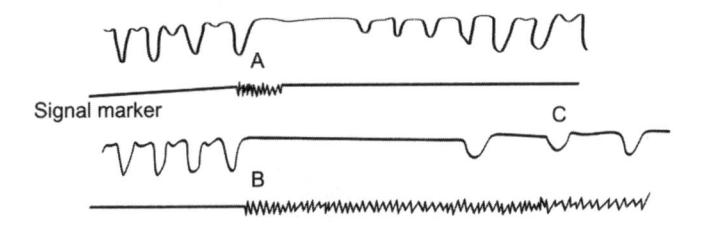

1. Explain the physiological basis of graphs A, B and C.
2. Why is the graph showing stimulation of the vagus and the white crescentic line similar?
3. How do you identify the vagus in the experimental preparation?
4. What types of fibers are carried by the vagus nerve?
5. What is the effect of continuous stimulation of the vagus and why?
6. What types of fibers are present at the white cresentic line?
7. What is the nerve supply of the atria and ventricles of the human heart?
8. The graph is obtained on stimulating the vagosympathetic trunk
   a. Explain the graph?
   b. What kind of fibers are present in the WCL. What is the effect of stimulating it?
9. The graph is obtained on stimulating the vagosympathetic trunk
   a. What will happen if the stimulation is continued?
   b. What is the neurotransmitter in the sympathetic?

i. Preganglionic fibers
ii. Postganglionic fibers.
10. The graph is obtained on stimulating an amphibian preparation
    a. What in your opinion has been stimulated?
    b. What kind of fibers does it carry?
    c. What is the neurotransmitter secreted at:
        i. Preganglionic sympathetic nerves
        ii. Postganglionic parasympathetic nerves.
11. Name the type of receptor at R1 and R2 and name the neurotransmitter secreted at them?

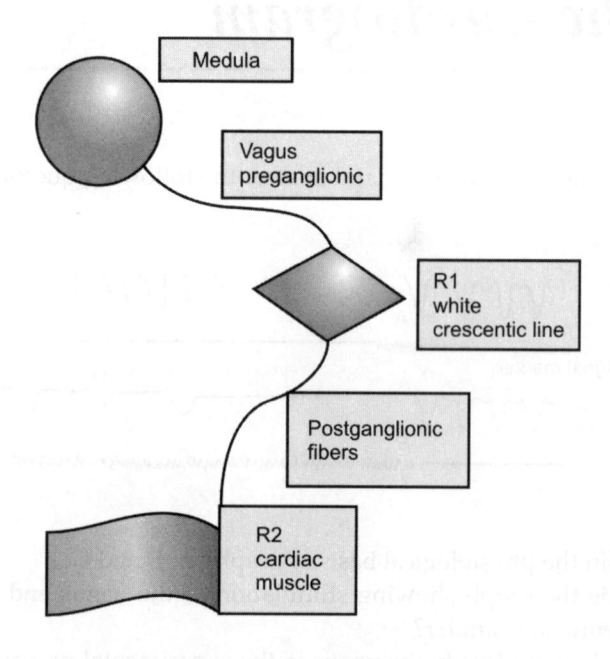

Chapter 29

Effect of Some Variables on the Isolated Frog's Heart and the Intact Frog's Heart

Study the graphs given below and answer the following questions.
1. Explain graphs (A to C).

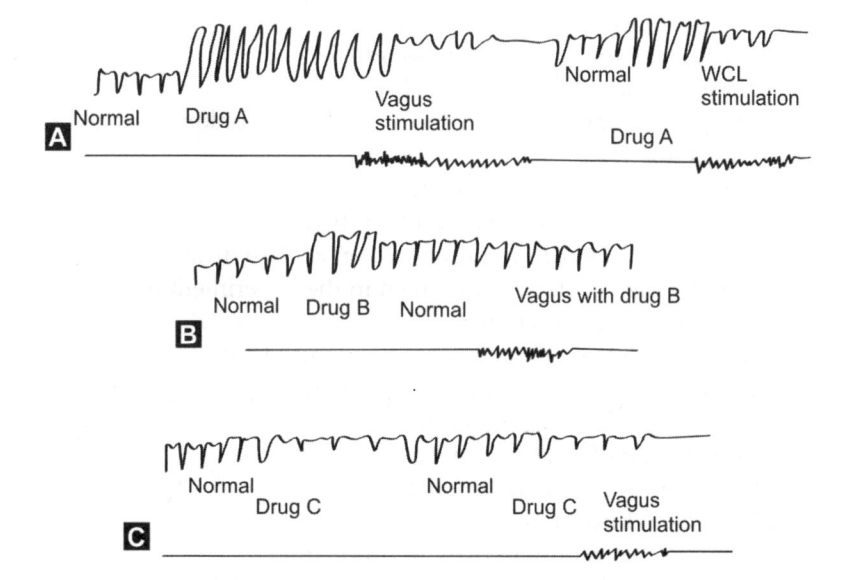

A Normal — Drug A — Vagus stimulation — Normal — WCL stimulation — Drug A

B Normal — Drug B — Normal — Vagus with drug B

C Normal — Drug C — Normal — Drug C — Vagus stimulation

2. Name two drugs that have negative ionotropic and chronotropic effect on the heart?
3. Name two drugs that have positive ionotropic and chronotropic effect on the heart?
4. How would you identify acetylcholine as an unknown drug?
5. How would you identify adrenalin as an unknown drug?
6. How would you identify nicotine as an unknown drug?
7. How would you identify atropine as an unknown drug?
8. What do you understand by the term chemical vagotomy?

9. Why is it important to stimulate both vagus and the white crescentric line to identify every unknown drug?
10. Give two differences in the functioning of the isolated and the intact heart?
11. Give two differences in the functioning of amphibian and mammalian heart?
12. In an isolated heart preparation, how can the perfusion pressure be increased?
13. What is the effect of adding NaCl on frog's heart rate and force of contraction?
14. What is the effect of adding KCl on the isolated heart?
15. What is the effect of adding calcium on frog's heart rate and force of contraction? If excess calcium is added what will be the effect and why?
16. The graph demonstrates the effect of adding an unknown drug A on the frog's heart.
    a. Identify the drug A?
    b. What is the mechanism of its action?
    c. Name one antagonist/blocker?
17. The graph demonstrates the effect of adding an unknown drug A on the frog's heart?
    a. Explain the effect of adding drug A?
    b. How can you prove the identity of drug A?
    c. Name one other drug/ion which can act like drug A?
18. Choose the correct steps undertaken in the experiment for recording the effect of an unknown drug.
    a. Record the effect of drugs on a stationary drum
    b. Record a normal cardiogram; stimulate vagosympathetic trunk (VST) and white crescentric line (WCL)
    c. Pour 1 drop of unknown drug
    d. Speed of drum should be 2.5 mm/sec
    e. Pour 2 - 3 drops of drug
    f. Increase the amount of drug to proceed on
    g. Stimulate the WCL but do not stimulate the VST after pouring the drug
    h. Stimulate the VST and WCL after adding the drug
    i. Stimulate the heart during early diastole.

COMMON QUESTION FOR EXPERIMENTAL

1. Identify the given instrument?
2. Mention one use of it?
3. Name the practicals in which it has been used?

Unit 3

Mammalian Experiments

30. Effect of Drugs on Movements of Small Intestine of Rabbit
31. Effect of Drugs and Variables on Perfusion of Isolated Heart of Rabbit

Chapter 30

Effect of Drugs on Movements of Small Intestine of Rabbit

QUESTION STATION

1. Why is the rabbit chosen for this experiment?
2. What portion of the intestine is dissected in this experiment?
3. What is the name of the solution used in this experiment?
4. Enumerate the constituents of the solution with their function?
5. What types of movements are recorded in the intestine?
6. Study the graph and identify the unknown drug?

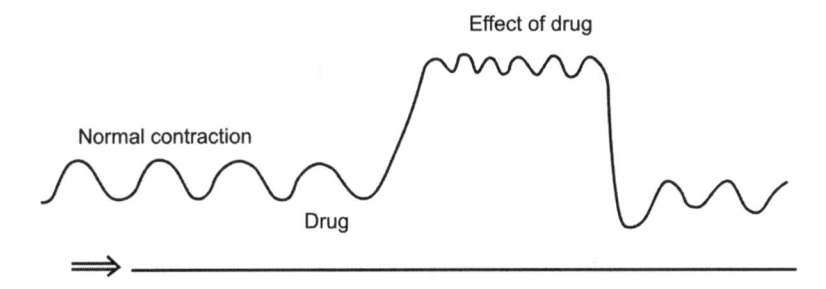

Effect of drug

Normal contraction

Drug

⇒

7. Name two drugs/ion which increase and two which decrease the activity of the small intestine?

Chapter 31

Effect of Drugs and Variables on Perfusion of Isolated Heart of Rabbit

QUESTION STATION

1. Name the apparatus used to see the effect of variables in isolated rabbit heart experiments?
2. Name the solution used to see the effect of variables in isolated rabbit heart experiments?
3. What is the need to continuously bubble oxygen into the preparation?
4. Can a similar experiment be done using a frog's heart?
5. At what pH is the solution kept?
6. What do you understand by the term perfusion pressure?
7. What is the effect of adrenalin on the heart rate and force of contraction?
8. A picture/diagram of an apparatus is shown to you. Identify and state what it is used for?

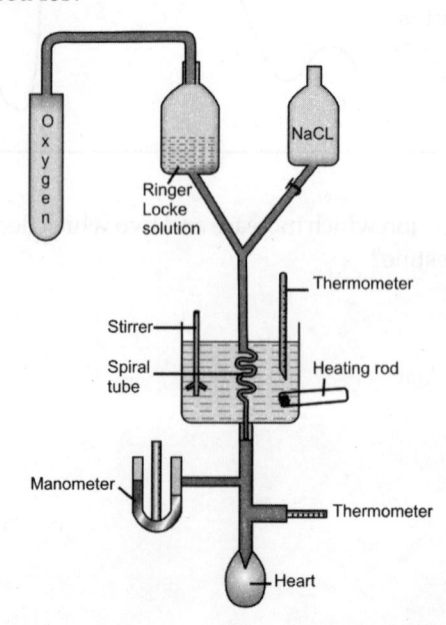

Effect of Drugs and Variables on Perfusion of Isolated Heart of Rabbit

9. A graph is placed in front of you. Identify the drug used?
10. Outline the path taken by the perfusate in this importance?
11. What is the normal perfusion pressure? If it is increased what would be the effect on the heart rate?
12. What is the physiological importance of knowing the perfusion pressure? How would you demonstrate the Frank Starling law using this preparation?
13. Name one sympathomimetic and one parasympathomimetic drug?
14. Enumerate two differences between the amphibian and the mammalian heart?

Unit 4

Human Experiments

32. Demonstration of Fatigue using Mosso's Ergograph
33. Recording of Systemic Arterial Blood Pressure
34. Effect of Posture on Blood Pressure
35. Effect of Exercise on Blood Pressure
36. Measurement of Blood Flow using Venous Occlusion Plethysmography
37. Recording of ECG
38. Effect of Exercise on Cardiovascular System
39. Study of Respiratory Movements by Stethography
40. Study of Lung Function by Spirometry
41. Effect of Posture on Vital Capacity
42. Effect of Exercise on the Respiratory System
43. Measurement of Basal Metabolic Rate
44. Determination of Mechanical Efficiency
45. Cardiopulmonary Resuscitation
46. Recording of Normal Body Temperature and Effect of Hot and Cold Environment on It
47. Semen Analysis
48. Pregnancy Diagnostic Tests
49. General Physical Examination
50. Clinical Examination of the Cardiovascular System
51. Clinical Examination of the Respiratory System
52. Clinical Examination of the Abdomen
53. Clinical Examination of the Sensory System
54. Clinical Examination of the Visual Acuity
55. Clinical Examination of Color Vision
56. Clinical Examination of the Eye by Retinoscopy and Ophthalmoscopy
57. Examination of Field of Vision by Perimetry
58. Clinical Examination of Cranial Nerve
59. Clinical Examination of Hearing
60. Clinical Examination of the Motor System
61. Clinical Examination of Higher Functions
62. Clinical Examination of Reflexes
63. Determination of Reaction Time
64. Electroencephalography
65. Evoked Potentials

Chapter 32

Demonstration of Fatigue using Mosso's Ergograph

QUESTION STATION

1. Work done was calculated using a Mosso's ergograph.
   a. Explain how venous occlusion is produced in this experiment?
   b. In which condition do you expect maximum work to be done?
      A= arterial occlusion   B= venous occlusion
   c. Enumerate two factors that can affect the onset of fatigue in man?
2. The diagram given below shows the work done by a student, using a Mosso's ergograph.

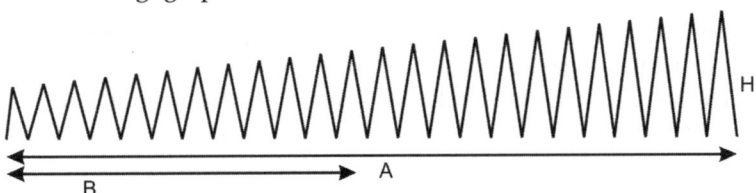

   a. Calculate the work done in normal circumstances (weight lifted = 2 kg)?
   b. What is the site of fatigue in:
      i. A frog's nerve muscle preparation
      ii. A human muscle.
3. The diagram shows an ergographic recording.
   a. Write down the formula for calculation of work done?
   b. Name two factors that influence the onset of fatigue?

4. Identify the instrument. What is it used for? What is the purpose of adding a greater weight to the experimental setup?

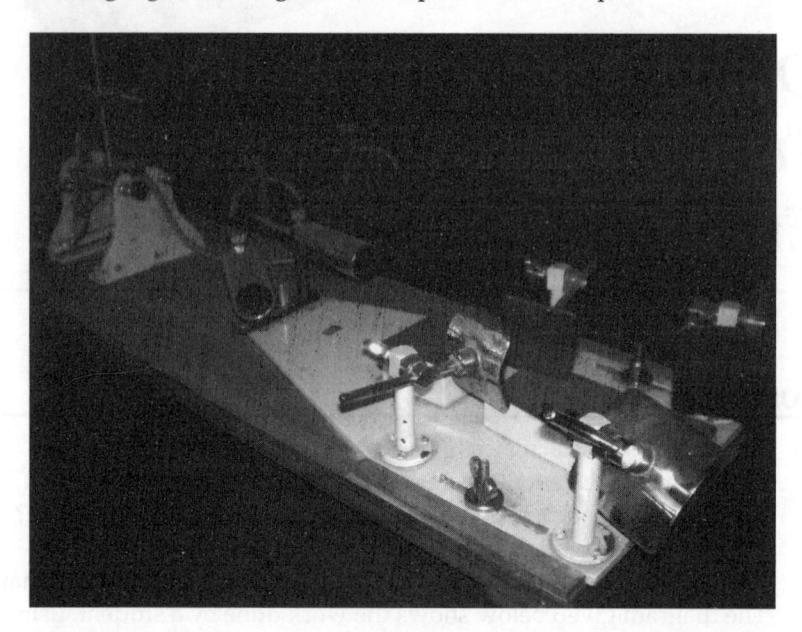

5. How do you decide about the frequency of finger movement?
6. How is the arterial occlusion brought about?
7. What is the difference between work done by venous and arterial occlusion?
9. Name two factors that can alter the time for onset of fatigue?
10. What is the site of fatigue in man?
11. Give the physiological reason for fatigue in a skeletal muscle?
12. Can the phenomenon of fatigue occur in:
    a. A smooth muscle
    b. Cardiac muscle.

Chapter 33

Recording of Systemic Arterial Blood Pressure

PROCEDURE STATION-1

Demonstrate the procedure of recording the blood pressure using a sphygmomanometer.

Checklist

1. Makes the subject comfortable.
2. Explains the procedure to him.
3. Deflates the cuff completely.
4. Ties the cuff correctly.
5. Raises the mercury about 200 mmHg for recording the systolic BP.
6. Lets the mercury drop at adequate speed.
7. Takes more than one reading.
8. Reports the systolic BP correctly.
9. Reports the diastolic BP correctly.

PROCEDURE STATION-2

Tie the sphygmomanometer cuff for measurement of BP.

Checklist

1. Chooses the appropriate size of the cuff.
2. Ensures that the cuff is completely deflated.
3. Instructs the subject suitably.
4. Positions the subject appropriately.
5. Exposes the arm properly.
6. Places the cuff to cover the medial aspect of the arm.
7. Ensures that the lower border of the cuff is approximately two finger breadths above the cubital fossa.
8. Ensures that the tubing does not overlie the fossa.
9. Ensures that the cuff is neither too tight nor too loose.

PROCEDURE STATION-3

Find the systolic blood pressure by the palpatory method.

Checklist

1. Instructs the subject.
2. Positions him appropriately.
3. Ties the cuff properly.
4. Checks that the lock of the instrument is in the "on" position.
5. Feels the radial pulse.
6. Inflates the cuff feeling the pulse simultaneously.
7. Deflates the cuff correctly, feeling the radial pulses simultaneously.
8. Records the systolic BP correctly.

PROCEDURE STATION-4

Find out the blood pressure by the auscultatory method given that the B.P. is 120/80 mm Hg by the palpatory method.

Checklist

1. Instructs the subject.
2. Positions him appropriately.
3. Ties the cuff properly.
4. Checks that the lock of the instrument is in the "on" position.
5. Positions the earpiece of the sthethoscope properly.
6. Checks that the diaphragm is in the "on" position.
7. Places the diaphragm of the stethoscope correctly so as to cover the brachial artery.
8. Inflates the cuff appropriately.
9. Deflates the cuff at appropriate speed.
10. Reports the BP correctly.
11. Ensures that the cuff is completely deflated at the end of the procedure.

QUESTION STATION

1. Enumerate the errors in the following passage:
   A subject's BP was recorded for the first time, as 120/181 mmHg, although the instrument at the beginning of the experiment showed a mercury column of 10 mm Hg. Based on this finding, treatment was started immediately.
   Checklist
   a. BP charting (0.2 each)
   b. Systolic/diastolic

c. Even no. of BP.
   d. Units
   e. Zero error.
2. Explain the cardiovascular reflex responsible for the same.
3. What is the normal range of BP in an adult?
4. What do you understand by the term auscultatory gap?
5. What is the principle of recording the BP by the auscultatory method?

Chapter 34

Effect of Posture on Blood Pressure

PROCEDURE STATION

Demonstrate the procedure of recording the effect of change of posture (from lying to standing position) on the blood pressure of the subject provided.

Checklist

1. Instructs the subject properly.
2. Makes him comfortable.
3. Takes the blood pressure in the lying position.
4. Records both the systolic and the diastolic blood pressure.
5. Takes more than one reading.
6. Lets the cuff remain on the arm.
7. Records the blood pressure in the standing position within 30 seconds.
8. Records both the systolic and the diastolic blood pressure again.
9. Records both pressures once again to see if they have changed from initial reading in the standing position.

QUESTION STATION

The blood pressure was recorded in the right arm of a subject in both the lying position and then immediately in the standing position.
1. What change do you expect in the BP immediately on standing in:
   a. Systolic BP
   b. Diastolic BP.

Chapter 35

Effect of Exercise on Blood Pressure

PROCEDURE STATION-1

Demonstrate the procedure of recording the changes in blood pressure with mild/moderate exercise.

Checklist

1. Instructs the subject properly.
2. Records the baseline blood pressure.
3. Lets the cuff remain on the arm of the subject while performing exercise.
4. Checks that the subject is performing the exercise procedure correctly.
5. Checks the blood pressure at regular intervals of the exercise.
6. Instructs the subject to stop exercise at the required time.
7. Checks the blood pressure at regular intervals of recovery.
8. Reports/Records correctly.

PROCEDURE STATION-2

Demonstrate the effect of exercise on systolic and diastolic BP.

Checklist

1. Instructs the subject.
2. Ties the cuff properly.
3. Checks the procedure of the exercise.
4. Records systolic BP
    a. Before
    b. Immediately after
    c. At fixed interval of time
    d. During recovery.
5. Records diastolic BP
    a. Before
    b. Immediately after
    c. At fixed interval of time
    d. During recovery.

QUESTION STATION

1. What is moderate exercise?
2. What changes do you expect in the diastolic and the systolic blood pressure with moderate exercise?
3. Explain your answer in the above question?
4. Should hypertensive patients be advised to exercise? Explain your answer?
5. What is the effect of mild exercise on the systolic and diastolic BP?
6. What is the effect of severe exercise on the systolic and diastolic BP?

Chapter 36

Measurement of Blood Flow using Venous Occlusion Plethysmography

PROCEDURE STATION-1

Demonstrate the procedure of calibrating the volume recorder to be used in venous occlusion plethysmography.

Checklist

1. Fills the volume recorder with water.
2. Balances it by adjusting the screws on the weight.
3. Checks that the pointer writes horizontally on the kymograph.
4. Fills a syringe with 10 ml of air.
5. Clamps the tube connected to the plethysmograph.
6. Injects the air into the instrument.
7. Marks the point of rise of the lever.
8. Repeats the procedure till calibration is complete.
9. Now clamps the calibration tube.

PROCEDURE STATION-2

Demonstrate the procedure of recording blood flow to the forearm using plethysmograph (BP of subject is given).

Checklist

1. Adjusts the speed of the kymograph (2.5 mm/sec).
2. Adjusts the time marker.
3. Checks for calibration.
4. Puts his forearm into the plethysmograph.
5. Adjusts the plethysmograph.
6. Ties the cuff of the sphygmomanometer on the upper arm.
7. Raises the pressure to 10 - 15 mm Hg below the diastolic pressure of the subject.
8. Waits for 30 seconds for the pointer to rise.

9. Stops the drum.
10. Records the volume change per unit time.

QUESTION STATION

Study the graph given below:
1. Calculate the blood flow of the forearm?
2. What two factors can influence the results?
3. Name one new technique that records blood flow to an organ?
4. State the physiological relevance of knowing blood flow through an organ?

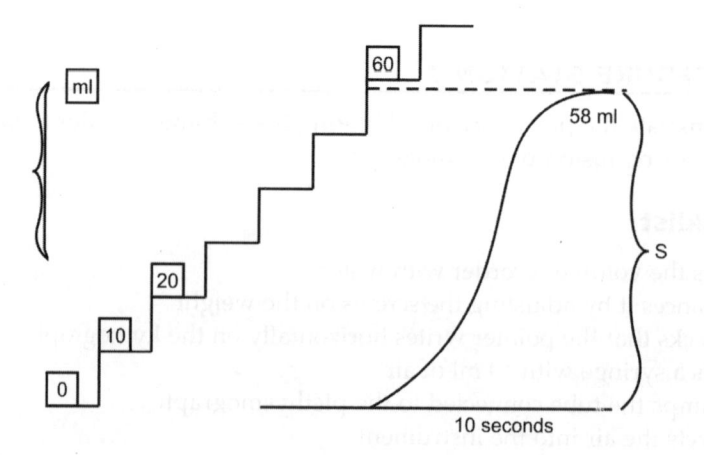

Chapter 37

Recording of ECG

1. A strip of ECG is provided to you.

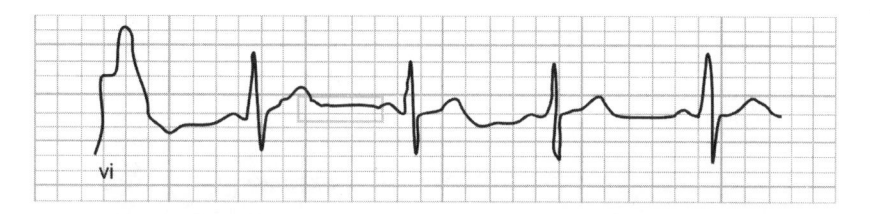

    a. Identify the lead.
    b. Mark the significant waves.
    c. Calculate PR, QT, ST interval.
    d. Mark the J point.
    e. Comment upon it.
    f. Calculate the heart rate?
    g. Name two indications of doing ECG in patients?
    h. What all information can you get from it?
    i. Draw an ECG with similar heart rate and first degree heart block?
2. An ECG with an abnormal finding is shown to you.
    a. Identify the abnormality?
    b. What complains is the patient likely to have?
    c. What should be the next line of management?

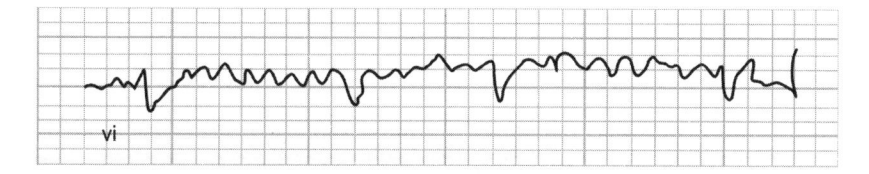

3. An instrument is placed in front of you.

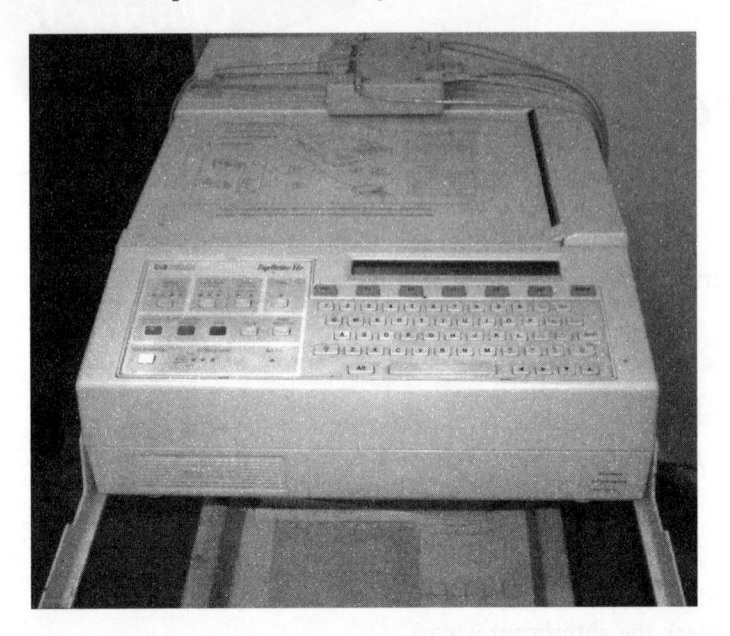

   a. Identify the instrument?
   b. Name two prerequisites that are essential before beginning the investigation?
   c. What is the routine speed of the instrument?
4. Draw a normal ECG in lead II?
5. Draw a normal ECG in aVR?

Chapter 38
Effect of Exercise on Cardiovascular System

PROCEDURE STATION

Demonstrate the procedure of recording the changes in heart rate with mild/moderate exercise.

Checklist

1. Instructs the subject properly.
2. Records the baseline parameters.
3. Checks that the subject is performing the exercise procedure correctly.
4. Checks the heart/pulse rate at regular intervals of the exercise.
5. Instructs the subject to stop exercise at the required time.
6. Checks the heart/pulse rate at regular intervals of recovery.
7. Reports/Record correctly.

QUESTION STATION

1. Name two precautions you would undertake before beginning the exercise?
2. Name two indications for stopping the exercise before time?
3. Name a clinical condition where exercise testing is used for diagnostic purposes?
4. Mention two changes that you expect in the cardiovascular system in mild/moderate/severe exercise?
5. What do you understand by the term MET?
6. Mention two changes that you expect in the respiratory system in mild/moderate/severe exercise?

Chapter 39
Study of Respiratory Movements by Stethography

PROCEDURE STATION

Record the effect of normal respiratory movements by stethography.

Checklist

1. Makes the subject comfortable.
2. Makes the subject sit with his/her back to the recording apparatus.
3. Ties the corrugated tube on the subject at appropriate site.
4. The tube is neither too tight nor too loose.
5. The connecting tube is connected to the Marey's tambour.
6. The time marker is adjusted.
7. The lever with the Mareys tambour marker is kept in the same level.
8. Starts the Kymograph at slow speed.
9. Takes appropriate recording.
10. Takes a time tracing.

QUESTION STATION

1. The graph showing recordings during different phases of a stethographic recording is shown.
    a. Identify phases A and B?
    b. What happens to the breath-holding time after deep inspiration compared with a normal expiration?
    c. Define Cheyne-Stroke breathing?
2. The graph showing recordings during different phases of a stethographic recording is shown.
    a. What is the breath holding time after inspiration?
    b. Identify phases A and B?
    c. What is the importance of using a corrugated rubber tubing in this experiment?

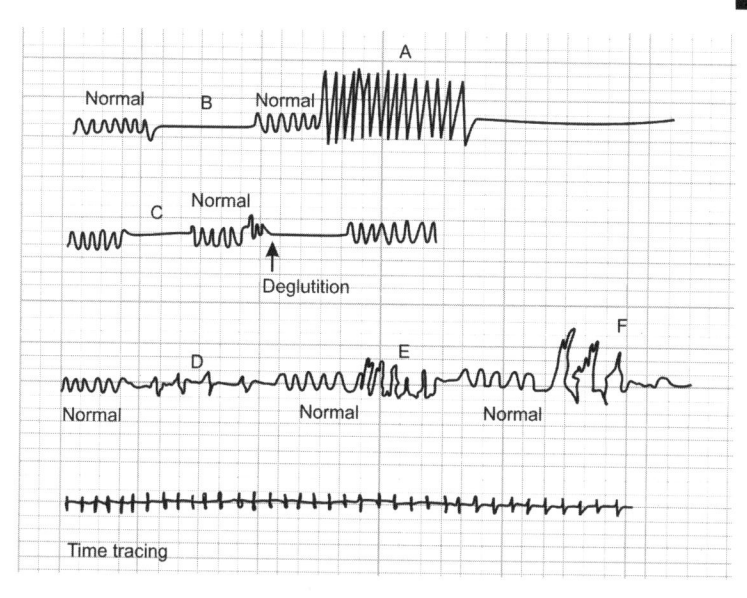

Study of Respiratory Movements by Stethography

3. One instrument is placed before you. It records some important physiological variables.
   a. Identify the instrument?

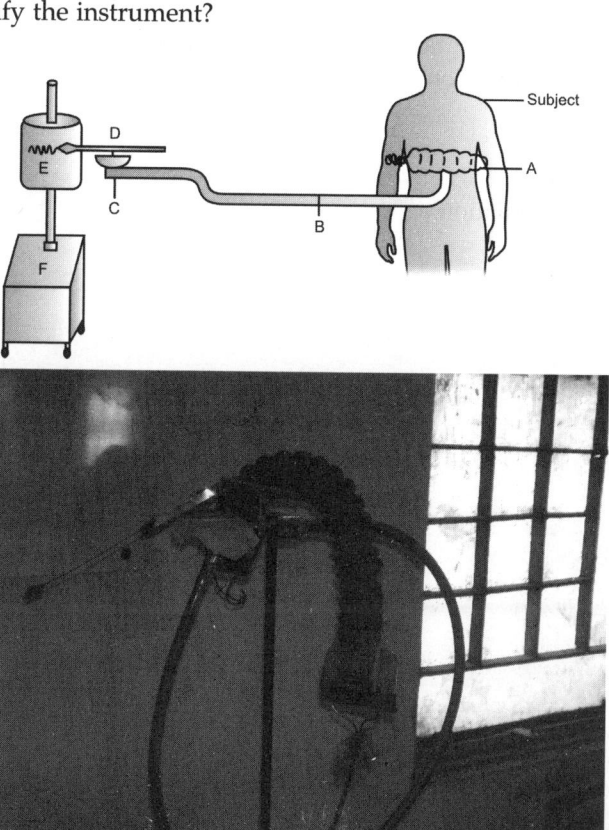

b. What are the variables that you can record using this instrument?
c. What is the physiological importance of the information that you can get from its recordings?
4. The various phases of respiration are recorded using a stethographic recording?
   a. In which phase of respiration is deglutination recorded?
   b. Explain the sequence of events following hyperventilation?
5. The stethographic recording is shown below:
   a. Calculate the breath holding time following inspiration?
   b. Enumerate conditions which lead to an increase in breath holding time?
   c. Explain the term Cheyne-Stroke respiration?
6. The graph shows breath holding time recorded during a stethographic recording.
   a. Calculate the breath holding time after inspiration?
   b. Can you prolong the duration of breath-holding? Explain your answer.
   c. Define "breaking point?"
   d. Identify phases A and B?
   e. What is the importance of using a corrugated rubber tubing in this experiment?
7. Draw a labeled diagram to show stethographic recording of:
   a. Normal respiration
   b. Talking
   c. Coughing
   d. Sneezing
   e. Hyperventillation.

Chapter 40
Study of Lung Function by Spirometry

PROCEDURE STATION-1

Demonstrate the procedure of recording the tidal volume of a subject with a spirometer.

Checklist

1. Instruct the subject correctly about the apparatus and the procedure.
2. Make the subject comfortable.
3. Instruct the subject to put the mouth piece in the mouth.
4. Ask the subject to inhale the atmospheric air in the room.
5. Ask the subject to exhale into the spirometer.
6. Take a fairly long record.

PROCEDURE STATION-2

Demonstrate the procedure of recording the inspiratory reserve volume, expiratory reserve volume, inspiratory and expiratory capacity of a subject with a spirometer.

Checklist

1. Instructs the subject correctly about the apparatus and the procedure.
2. Makes the subject comfortable.
3. Instructs the subject to put the mouth piece in the mouth.
4. Asks the subject to inhale the atmospheric air in the room.
5. Asks the subject to exhale into the spirometer.
6. Takes a fairly long record.
7. Takes a normal inspiration and expiration.
8. After a normal expiration breathes in maximally.
9. Subtracts the normal tidal volume from this to get the inspiratory reserve volume.
10. After 7 Breathes out maximally and records this.
11. Subtracts the tidal volume from this total for the expiratory reserve volume.
12. Record 8 as inspiratory capacity and 10 as expiratory capacity.

QUESTION STATION

From the record of the spirometric tracing:

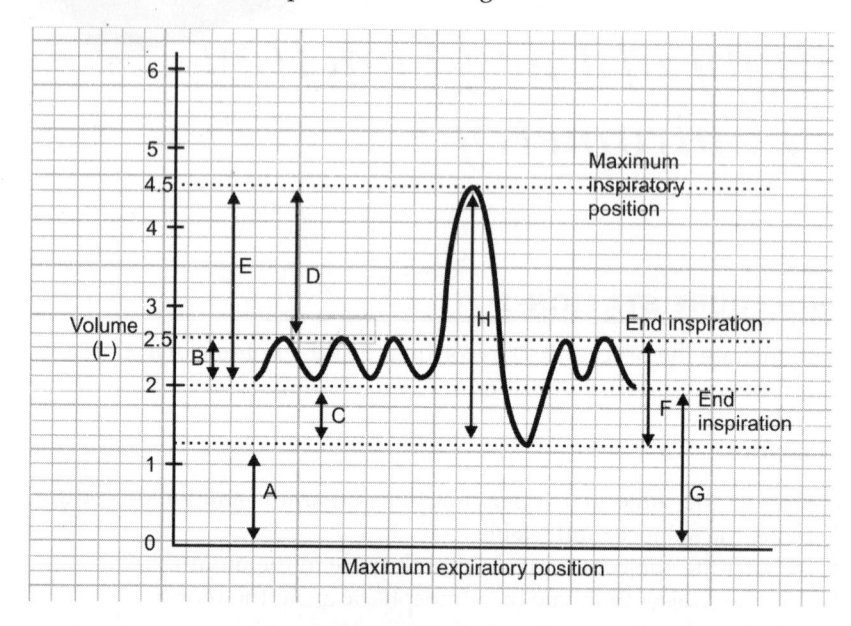

1. Calculate the inspiratory capacity?
2. Calculate the inspiratory reserve volume?
3. Calculate the expiratory reserve volume?
4. Calculate the total lung capacity?
5. Calculate the FEV_1?
6. Calculate the FEV_2?
7. Calculate the vital capacity?
8. What is the ratio of FEV_1/VC in normal and asthmatic lung?
9. Identify the instrument (Peak flow meter)

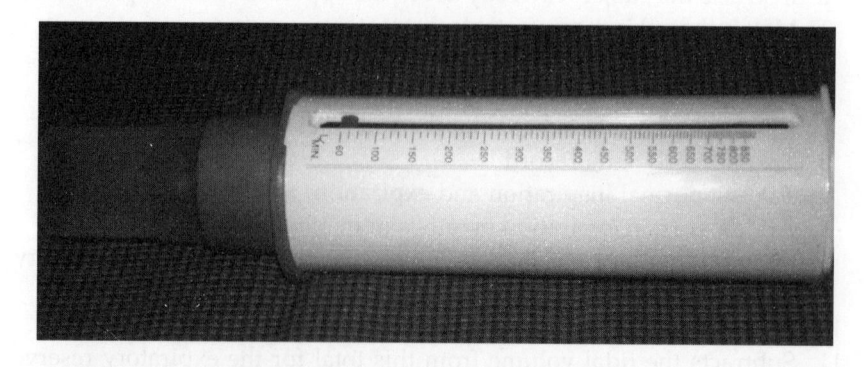

Chapter 41

Effect of Posture on Vital Capacity

PROCEDURE STATION

Demonstrate the procedure of recording the effect of posture on vital capacity.

Checklist

1. Instructs the subject.
2. Makes him comfortable.
3. Records vital capacity in the three postures (sitting, standing, supine).
4. Takes more than one reading for each.
5. Reports correctly.

QUESTION STATION

1. Define "vital capacity?"
2. Name the posture where the vital capacity is maximum?
3. Name two conditions in which the vital capacity decreases?
4. Enumerate two physiological conditions when vital capacity is more?

Chapter 42

Effect of Exercise on the Respiratory System

PROCEDURE STATION

Demonstrate the procedure of recording changes in the respiratory system after mild-moderate exercise.

Checklist

1. Instructs the subject.
2. Makes him comfortable.
3. Records respiratory rate in standing position.
4. Records the tidal volume in the standing position.
5. Makes the subject do exercise.
6. After the exercise records respiratory rate in standing position.
7. After the exercise records tidal volume in standing position.
8. Timing of recording postexercise events is appropriate.

QUESTION STATION

1. Why should the respiratory rate change with exercise?
2. What changes occur in the respiratory volume with exercise?
3. Name the respiratory variable whose measurement gives you an indication about the severity of exercise?

Chapter 43

Measurement of Basal Metabolic Rate

PROCEDURE STATION

Demonstrate the procedure of measurement of resting metabolic rate at body temperature.

Checklist

1. Instructs the subject.
2. Makes the subject comfortable.
3. Checks that the spirometer is filled with 100% oxygen.
4. Connects the subject to the apparatus.
5. Tells the subject to breathe in atmospheric air for sometime.
6. Now connects the subject to the spirometer.
7. The subject breathes in and out of the apparatus.

QUESTION STATION

1. Identify the use of the instrument if it contains oxygen?
2. At what temperatures can the recordings be made?
3. Write the formula used to make calculations for the parameter tested using this instrument?
4. The instrument provided or shown to you is used to measure the basal metabolic rate:
   a. What is basal metabolic rate and what is resting metabolic rate?
   b. Name two factors which determine the basal metabolic rate?
   c. Name two factors which affect the basal metabolic rate?
5. The volume of oxygen consumed per minute at BPTS is 2 liters in 6 minutes:
   a. Find out the volume of oxygen consumed per minute at BPTS?
   b. Find out the heat production at RQ of 0.8?
6. From the normograms provided find out:
   a. The expected BMR of the subject?
   b. The surface area of the 25 years old male subject of height 170 cm and weighing 60 Kg?

Chapter 44

Determination of Mechanical Efficiency

QUESTION STATION

1. What do you understand by the term steady state?
2. Calculate the external work done if a person weighing 60 Kg moves the wheels of a cycle for a distance of 2 km with a tension load of 2 Kg?
3. Calculate the mechanical efficiency of 40 Kilopond meter work done, if 2.5 liters of oxygen is consumed at STPD (1 Kilo cal = 426.7 Kpm/min)?

Chapter 45

Cardiopulmonary Resuscitation

PROCEDURE STATION

Demonstrate the procedure of doing cardiac massage in a dummy.

Checklist

1. Exposes the chest of the dummy provided.
2. Selects the site (upper 2/3 and lower 1/3 sternum).
3. Places the heel of his hand on the site.
4. Places the heel of the second hand over the first.
5. Position of the hand is satisfactory (fingers should not be touching).
6. Position of the elbow is satisfactory (elbow is straight).
7. Pushes one hand over the other.
8. Force of the hand is vertically downward.
9. Movement of the arm occurs at the shoulders.
10. The sternum is compressed about 4 - 5 cm.
11. Rate of compression is about 70 - 80/minute.

QUESTION STATION

1. Mention the first prerequisite to begin resuscitation of a subject?
2. What is the rate of artificial breathing to be induced?
3. At what rate must the cardiac massage be given?
4. How is expiration brought about?
5. How long must cardiopulmonary resuscitation continue in a patient?
6. What difference must be kept in mind while doing cardiac massage of an infant as compared to an adult?

Chapter 46

Recording of Normal Body Temperature and Effect of Hot and Cold Environment on It

PROCEDURE STATION-1

Demonstrate the procedure of recording the temperature in the subject provided.

Checklist

1. Instructs the subject (not to bite, lips held closely around).
2. Makes him comfortable.
3. Takes a clinical thermometer.
4. Shakes it to bring down the mercury column.
5. Inserts the bulb of the thermometer into the subject's mouth.
6. The bulb is placed beneath the tongue.
7. Keeps the thermometer there for a minute.
8. Takes the thermometer out.
9. Reads it.
10. Reports correctly.
11. Cleans the thermometer(puts it in savlon etc.).

PROCEDURE STATION-2

Demonstrate the procedure of recording the skin temperature at various sites in the subject provided.

Checklist

1. Instructs the subject (not to bite, lips held closely around).
2. Makes him comfortable.
3. Takes a clinical thermometer.
4. Shakes it to bring down the mercury column.

5. Puts thermometer at the following sites (palm, back of hand, fingers, forehead, back, axilla, sternum, dorsum of foot.
6. Fixes the thermometer in each of this position with a leucoplast.
7. Leaves the thermometer in each site for atleast a minute.
8. Report each correctly (mark distribution should be such, that 5, 6, 7 to be given more weightage).

Chapter 47

Semen Analysis

PROCEDURE STATION-1

Demonstrate the procedure of preparing the hanging drop preparation of the semen sample.

Checklist

1. Takes a clean slide.
2. Takes plasticine and rolls it to form a ring.
3. A thin ring is formed.
4. Puts the ring on the slide.
5. Takes the sample (diluted/not diluted) in a test tube.
6. Takes a wire loop or a dropper to take a drop of the sample.
7. Takes a cover slip and puts a drop of the sample on it.
8. Holds the slide with plasticine facing downward.
9. Puts the slide on the cover slip, such that it seals the drop of semen forming a hanging drop preparation.
10. Reverses the preparation such that the slide is at the bottom and the cover slip is on top.
11. Places it under the low power of the microscope to visualize.

PROCEDURE STATION-2

Demonstrate the procedure of doing the sperm count for analysis.

Checklist

1. Wears gloves.
2. Takes the sample provided in a test tube, placed in a rack.
3. Checks for dilution if any.
4. Gently shakes the sample.
5. Takes the WBC pipette.
6. Draws semen in the tube till the 0.5 mark.
7. Draws dilution fluid (4% sodium bicarbonate solution in 1% phenol solution) till mark 11.
8. Rolls the pipette.
9. Discards 1 - 2 drops.

10. Charges the chamber.
11. Counts the sperms in high power.
12. WBC counting area is exposed.

QUESTION STATION

1. Write what you would expect in a normal semen analysis report?
2. Draw a normal human sperm labeling it?
3. Draw four abnormal morphological patterns of sperms?
4. How would you describe the motility of a normal sperm?
5. How would you grade the motility of a sperm?
6. Name two patterns of abnormal motility?

Chapter 48

Pregnancy Diagnostic Tests

PROCEDURE STATION

Demonstrate the procedure of doing the immunological test for diagnosing pregnancy.

Checklist

1. Takes few ml of the sample urine.
2. Takes a control sample.
3. Adds reagent/s to the wells.
4. Puts both in separate wells.
5. Looks for agglutination/color change.
6. Reports correctly.
7. Wears gloves.

QUESTION STATION

1. Match the following:

Sample injected	Animal	Name of test
A. 2 ml urine s/c	Female Immature mice	a. Aschheim-Zondak test
B. 2 ml urine s/c	Female Immature rats	b. Kuppermann test
C. 10 - 15 ml urine IV	Female rabbit	c. Friedman test
D. 20 - 30 ml urine in dorsal lymph sac	Female toad	d. Hogben test
E. Urine	Male frog	e. Galli-Mainini test

2. The immunological test for pregnancy is routinely carried out.
   a. What is it that you test for in a urine sample of a pregnant patient?
   b. Name a condition that gives a false positive test for pregnancy?
   c. What is the least duration of pregnancy for which this test is positive?
   d. What is the hormone whose presence and increased level indicates pregnancy?
   e. What is the minimum level of the hormone mentioned above?

Chapter 49

General Physical Examination

PROCEDURE STATION-1

Demonstrate the procedure of examining the stature of the subject.

Checklist

1. Instructs the subject.
2. Makes him comfortable.
3. Asks the subject to stand straight and erect without shoes against a wall.
4. Measures his height using a vertical scale.
5. Makes the subject stand on a weighing machine using indoor clothings without shoes.
6. Records his weight.
7. Calculates the body mass index.
8. Measures the girth, midway between the costal margin and the iliac crest.
9. Looks for abnormal fat distribution.
10. Looks for malnourishment and signs of vitamin deficiency.
11. Reports correctly.

PROCEDURE STATION-2

Demonstrate the procedure of taking temperature of the subject.

Checklist

1. Instructs the subject.
2. Makes him comfortable.
3. Takes a clinical thermometer.
4. Cleans the bulb.
5. Shakes the thermometer so that the mercury falls.
6. Puts the thermometer under the subjects tongue.
7. Keeps it there for at least 30 seconds.
8. Takes it out and notes the reading.

9. Reports correctly.
10. Puts it back in the antiseptic solution.

PROCEDURE STATION-3

Demonstrate the procedure of recording the respiratory rate of the subject.

Checklist

1. Instructs the subject.
2. Makes him comfortable.
3. Exposes the abdomen of the subject.
4. Checks that the respiratory movements are uniform.
5. Waits for some time for the respiratory movements and the rate to become uniform.
6. Counts the rate visually without making the subject conscious.
7. Counts for at least 30 seconds.
8. Reports correctly.
9. Covers or instructs the subject to cover his/her abdomen.

PROCEDURE STATION-4

Demonstrate the procedure of checking for pallor of the subject.

Checklist

1. Instructs the subject.
2. Makes him comfortable.
3. Gently lowers the lower eyelid to check for pallor.
4. Checks the pallor in both eyes.
5. Looks at the nail bed.
6. Reports correctly.

PROCEDURE STATION-5

Demonstrate the procedure of checking for edema of the subject.

Checklist

1. Instructs the subject.
2. Makes him comfortable.
3. Exposes the region above the medial malleolus near the ankle.
4. Presses the area for about 30 seconds.
5. Looks for oedema in the other limb/dependant areas.
6. Reports correctly.

PROCEDURE STATION-6

Demonstrate the procedure of checking the JVP of the subject.

Checklist

1. Instructs the subject.
2. Makes him comfortable.
3. Positions the patient in the lying position with the neck bent.
4. Reports correctly.

PROCEDURE STATION-7

Demonstrate the procedure of examining the cervical lymph nodes of the subject.

Checklist

1. Instructs the subject.
2. Seats him comfortably.
3. Inspects for any visible lymphadenopathy.
4. Stands behind the patient.
5. Using both hands palpates the anterior triangle of the neck (for submental, submandibular, preauricular, tonsillar, supraclavicular, deep cervical).
6. Palpates the scalene nodes with index finger in the angle between the sternocleidomastoid.
7. Now stands in front of the patient.
8. Palpates for glands in the posterior triangle.
9. Palpates for nodes up the back of neck, posterior auricular and occipital nodes.
10. Reports for site, size, consistency, tenderness, fixing of nodes.

PROCEDURE STATION-8

Demonstrate the procedure of examining the axillary lymph nodes of the subject.

Checklist

1. Instructs the subject.
2. Seats him comfortably.
3. Inspects for any visible lymphadenopathy.
4. Stands infront of the patient.
5. Supports the arm on the side to be examined.
6. Palpates the right axilla with the left hand and vice versa.

7. Feels the anterior, posterior, medial and axillary walls in turn.
8. Reports for site, size, consistency, tenderness, fixing of nodes.

PROCEDURE STATION-9

Demonstrate the procedure of examining the epitrochlear lymph nodes of the subject.

Checklist

1. Instruct the subject.
2. Seat him comfortably.
3. Inspect for any visible lymphadenopathy.
4. Stand infront of the patient
5. Support the patients right wrist with left hand and viceversa.
6. Grasp the patients partially flexed elbow with the ipsilateral hand.
7. Feel for epitrochlear LN with ipsilateral hand.
8. Report for site, size, consistency, tenderness, fixing of nodes.

PROCEDURE STATION-10

Demonstrate the procedure of examining the inguinal lymph nodes of the subject.

Checklist

1. Instructs the subject.
2. Seats him comfortably.
3. Inspects for any visible lymphadenopathy.
4. Stands in front of the patient.
5. Exposes the lower limb.
6. Palpates for the horizontal chain below the inguinal ligament.
7. Palpates for the vertical chain along the line of saphenous vein.
8. Reports for site, size, consistency, tenderness, fixing of nodes.

Chapter 50
Clinical Examination of the Cardiovascular System

PROCEDURE STATION-1

Demonstrate the procedure of taking the pulse of the subject provided.

Checklist

1. Instructs the subject and makes him comfortable.
2. Positions his hand properly.
3. Places three fingers on the radial pulse.
4. Records the pulse for atleast 30 sec.
5. Records the pulse atleast two different sites.
6. Reports the finding correctly.

PROCEDURE STATION-2

Demonstrate the procedure of recording the apex beat.

Checklist

1. Instructs the subject and makes him comfortable.
2. Exposes the part to be examined.
3. Counts the ribs.
4. Looks for the midclavicular line.
5. Finds the apex beat (asks patient to roll over if required).
6. Palpates it for 30 sec.
7. Confirms it with a stethoscope.

PROCEDURE STATION-3

Demonstrate the procedure of examination of the venous system.

Checklist

1. Instructs the subject.
2. Makes him comfortable.
3. Examines the patient's limb with the patient standing.

4. Examines the patient's limb with the patient supine.
5. Exposes the limb.
6. Examines the skin for color, swelling, superficial venous dilatation and tourtous veins.
7. Feels for any difference in temperature.
8. Elevates the limb for 15 degree above the horizontal and notes the rate of venous emptying.
9. May perform the trendelenburg test to look for saphenofemoral junction incompetence.

PROCEDURE STATION-4

Demonstrate the procedure of doing the Trendelenburg test.

Checklist

1. Instructs the subject.
2. Makes him comfortable.
3. Asks the subject to sit at the edge of the examination couch.
4. Elevates the limb till it is comfortable for the subject.
5. Empties the superficial vein by 'milking'.
6. Presses the thumb/puts a tourniquet over the saphenofemoral junction.
7. Now asks the patient to stand.
8. Looks for filling of the varicose veins.
9. Reports correctly.

PROCEDURE STATION-5

Demonstrate the procedure of examining the JVP.

Checklist

1. Instructs the subject.
2. Makes him comfortable.
3. Positions the patient reclining at 45° in good light.
4. Relaxes the neck muscles by resting back of the head on a pillow.
5. Stands on the right side of the patient.
6. Looks at the neck.
7. Identifies the internal jugular pulsation (May use abdominojugular reflex).
8. Finds the vertical height between the sternal angle and the top of venous pulsation.
9. Reports correctly.

PROCEDURE STATION-6

Demonstrate the examining of all the pulses.

Checklist

1. Instructs the subject.
2. Makes him comfortable.
3. Examines the radial pulse.
4. Examines the brachial pulse.
5. Examines the carotid pulse.
6. Examines the femoral pulse.
7. Examines the popliteal pulse.
8. Examines the posterior tibial pulse.
9. Examines the dorsalis pedis pulse.

PROCEDURE STATION-7

Demonstrate the procedure of examining the Brachial pulse of the subject.

Checklist

1. Instructs the subject.
2. Makes him comfortable.
3. Exposes the cubital fossa area (arm and forearm).
4. Uses the right thumb for the right arm and same for the other arm.
5. Supports the arm by cupping it with the fingers of the other hand.
6. Feels medial to the tendon of the biceps.
7. Feels for at least 30 seconds.
8. Reports correctly.

PROCEDURE STATION-8

Demonstrate the procedure of examining the carotid pulse of the subject.

Checklist

1. Instructs the subject.
2. Makes him comfortable.
3. Subjects should be lying on the bed.
4. Uses the left thumb for the right carotid artery and vice versa.
5. Places the thumb between the larynx and the anterior border of the sternocleidomastoid.
6. Feels the pulse.
7. Listens for bruits over the artery using the bell of a stethoscope.

PROCEDURE STATION-9

Demonstrate the procedure of examining the chest for heart sounds of the subject.

Checklist

1. Instructs the subject.
2. Makes him comfortable.
3. Asks the subject to remove clothing upto the waist.
4. Makes the patient lie 45° to the horizontal.
5. Listens over the precordium at the base of the heart, apex, upper left and right sternal edges.
6. Listens with both the bell and the diaphragm.
7. Listens over the carotid arteries and the axilla.
8. Rolls the patient on the left side.
9. Listens with the bell pressed slightly over the apex.
10. Sits the patient up and forward.
11. Asks the subject to breathe out completely and to hold his breath.
12. Listens over the right second intercostal space and over the left sternal edge with the diaphragm.
13. Reports the character and intensity of the first and second heart sound.
14. Reports murmers, added sounds, splitting of the second heart sound.
15. Notes the intensity and the character of the murmer heard.

QUESTION STATION

1. The diagram shows the auscultatory areas of the precordium

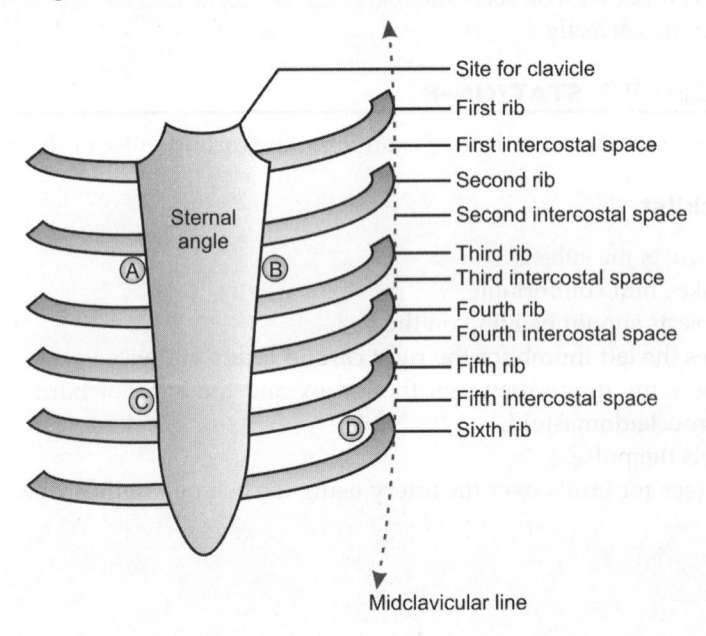

a. Name the areas A, B, C and D?
b. What are S3 and S4? Are they normally heard?
c. In which heart sound is the physiological split demonstrated?
2. The jugular venous pressure of a patient is measured and found to be high.
   a. What is the position of the patient in which JVP is measured?
   b. Give two differentiating features between arterial and venous pulsation?
   c. Name two conditions in which the jugular venous pressure is high?

Chapter 51
Clinical Examination of the Respiratory System

PROCEDURE STATION-1

Demonstrate the procedure of recording the vocal resonance of the subject provided.

Checklist

1. Instructs the subject and makes him comfortable.
2. Places the stethoscope at appropriate places.
3. Records in more than one area.
4. Reports correctly.

PROCEDURE STATION-2

Demonstrate the procedure of palpation of the respiratory system.

Checklist

1. Instructs the subject and makes him comfortable.
2. Checks for the position of trachea.
3. Checks for the vocal fremitus.
4. Checks for the bilateral expansion of the chest.
5. Reports correctly.

PROCEDURE STATION-3

Demonstrate the procedure of auscultation of the respiratory system.

Checklist

1. Instructs the subject and makes him comfortable.
2. Checks for breath sounds.
3. Checks for vocal resonance.
4. Checks in more than one area.
5. Reports correctly.

PROCEDURE STATION-4

Demonstrate the procedure of examining chest expansion of the respiratory system.

Checklist

1. Instructs the subject.
2. Makes him comfortable.
3. Exposes the chest.
4. Warms his hands.
5. Places his hand on the chest wall with thumbs meeting in the centre and fingers extending around the sides of the chest.
6. Asks the patient to take a deep breath. Looks for expansion (thumbs move apart by 5 cm).
7. Repeats in other areas from above downward.
8. Reports correctly.

PROCEDURE STATION-5

Demonstrate the procedure of percussion in the respiratory system.

Checklist

1. Instructs the subject.
2. Makes him comfortable.
3. Exposes the chest.
4. Warms his hands.
5. Places one hand with fingers slightly separated on the chest wall.
6. Presses the middle finger on the chest wall.
7. Strikes the centre of the middle phalanx with the tip of the right middle finger.
8. Movement should be from the wrist and not the forearm.
9. Percusses all the areas of the lung.
10. Percusses corresponding areas on the chest wall simultaneously.
11. Percusses the clavicle.
12. Moves from resonant to the dull area.
13. Reports correctly.

QUESTION STATION

1. Name the normal type of breath sounds?
2. Name two obstructive airway diseases. What is the type of breathing recorded in the disease?
3. What is the normal position of the trachea?
4. What additional precaution must be taken in examining the chest of a child?

Chapter 52

Clinical Examination of the Abdomen

PROCEDURE STATION-1

Demonstrate the procedure of palpating the spleen in the subject.

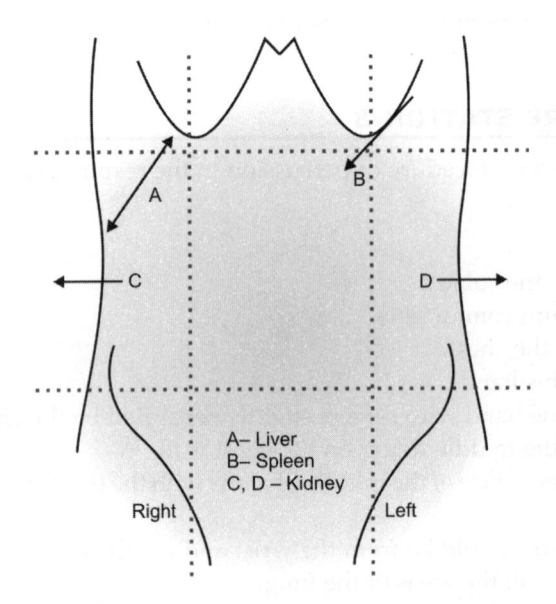

A– Liver
B– Spleen
C, D – Kidney

Right   Left

Checklist

1. Instructs the subject.
2. Makes him comfortable.
3. Exposes the abdomen of the subject.
4. Warms his hands.
5. Stands on the right side of the patient.
6. Places the left hand posterolaterally under the lowermost rib on the left side of the abdomen.
7. The right hand is placed below the right costal margin.
8. Asks the subject to breathe in deeply.

Clinical Examination of the Abdomen 111

9. At the height of inspiration presses right hand beneath the costal margin.
10. At the same time the left hand is pushing medially and downward.
11. Repeats with the right hand moving more medially beneath the costal margin.
12. Movement of the hand are smooth and not poking.
13. Reports correctly.

PROCEDURE STATION-2

Demonstrate the procedure of palpating the Liver in the subject.

Checklist

1. Instructs the subject.
2. Makes him comfortable.
3. Exposes the abdomen of the subject.
4. Warms his hands.
5. Stands on the right side of the patient.
6. Places both hands flatly on the abdomen in the right position.
7. Asks the subject to breathe in deeply.
8. At the height of inspiration presses fingers inwards and upwards.
9. Movements of the hand are smooth and not poking.
10. Reports correctly.

PROCEDURE STATION-3

Demonstrate the procedure of palpating the right kidney in the subject.

Checklist

1. Instructs the subject.
2. Makes him comfortable.
3. Exposes the abdomen of the subject.
4. Warms his hands.
5. Stands on the right side of the patient.
6. Places left hand posteriorly in the loin.
7. Places right hand in the right lumber region anteriorly.
8. Asks the subject to breathe in deeply.
9. At the height of inspiration presses right hand upwards and inwards and the left hand upwards.
10. Movements of the hand are smooth and not poking.
11. Reports correctly.

PROCEDURE STATION-4

Demonstrate the procedure of eliciting shifting dullness in the subject.

Checklist

1. Instructs the subject.
2. Makes him comfortable.
3. Exposes the abdomen of the subject.
4. Warms his hands.
5. Stands on the right side of the patient.
6. Places both hands as in percussion on the abdomen in the centre.
7. Starts percussing and then moves laterally till the dull note appears.
8. Asks the subject to roll over such that the lateral part of the abdomen now lies on top.
9. Percusses again, ensuring that his hand does not move away from the area.
10. Movements of the hand are smooth and not poking.
11. Reports correctly.

PROCEDURE STATION-5

Demonstrate the procedure of eliciting a fluid thrill in the subject.

Checklist

1. Instructs the subject.
2. Makes him comfortable.
3. Exposes the abdomen of the subject.
4. Warms his hands.
5. Stands on the right side of the patient.
6. Places one hand flatly on the side of the abdomen in the right position.
7. Asks the subject or an assistant to put the side of his hand in the midline.
8. Taps the other side of the abdomen
9. Movement of the hand are smooth and not poking.
10. Reports correctly.

PROCEDURE STATION-6

Demonstrate the procedure of defining the boundaries of liver.

Checklist

1. Instructs the subject.
2. Makes him comfortable.
3. Exposes the abdomen of the subject.
4. Warms his hands.

5. Stands on the right side of the patient.
6. Starts per cussing from the 4th intercostals space on the right side.
7. Moves downward to mark the upper border of liver.
8. Continues percussion to identify the lower border.
9. Movement of the hand are smooth and not poking.
10. Reports correctly.

Chapter 53

Clinical Examination of the Sensory System

PROCEDURE STATION-1

Demonstrate the procedure of testing fine touch in the subject provided.

Checklist

1. Instructs the subject.
2. Makes him comfortable.
3. Asks the subject to close his eyes.
4. Uses a fine wisp of cotton wool to test.
5. Moves along a particular dermatome.
6. Tests both the limb.
7. Reports correctly.

PROCEDURE STATION-2

Demonstrate the procedure of testing pressure sense in the subject provided.

Checklist

1. Instructs the subject.
2. Makes him comfortable.
3. Asks the subject to close his eyes.
4. Uses a blunt object at body temperature to test.
5. Moves along a particular dermatome.
6. Tests both the limb.
7. Reports correctly.

PROCEDURE STATION-3

Demonstrate the procedure of testing pain in the subject provided.

Checklist

1. Instructs the subject.
2. Makes him comfortable.
3. Asks the subject to close his eyes.

Clinical Examination of the Sensory System   115

4. Uses a common pin at body temperature to test.
5. Moves along a particular dermatome.
6. Tests both the limb.
7. Reports correctly.

PROCEDURE STATION-4

Demonstrate the procedure of testing deep pain in the subject provided.

Checklist

1. Instructs the subject.
2. Makes him comfortable.
3. Asks the subject to close his eyes.
4. Squeezes the muscle bellies (calf, bicep).
5. Applys pressure on the finger or toe nail bed.
6. Asks/looks for patient's response.
7. Maps out areas of reduced, absent or increased sensation.

PROCEDURE STATION-5

Demonstrate the procedure of testing temperature sense in the subject provided.

Checklist

1. Instructs the subject.
2. Makes him comfortable.
3. Asks the subject to close his eyes.
4. Uses test tubes containing hot and cold water alternately or randomly to test.
5. Moves along a particular dermatome.
6. Tests both the limb.
7. Reports correctly.

PROCEDURE STATION-6

Demonstrate the procedure of testing vibration sense in the subject provided.

Checklist

1. Instructs the subject.
2. Makes him comfortable.
3. Asks the subject to close his eyes.
4. Uses 128 Hz tuning fork to test.

5. Puts the foot of vibrating tuning fork on subcutaneous bone of limb. (sternum, tip of right toe, interphalangeal joint, medial malleolus, tibial tuberosity, anterior iliac spine, distal interphalangeal joint of the finger, radial styloid, olecranon, acromion).
6. Compares with the other limb when vibration stops.
7. Reports correctly.

PROCEDURE STATION-7

Demonstrate the procedure of testing position sense in the subject provided.

Checklist

1. Instructs the subject.
2. Makes him comfortable.
3. Asks the subject to close his eyes.
4. Moves his limb to a particular position.
5. Asks him to move the other corresponding limb in a similar position.
6. Reports correctly.

PROCEDURE STATION-8

Demonstrate the procedure of testing two point discrimination in the subject provided.

Checklist

1. Instructs the subject.
2. Makes him comfortable.
3. Asks the subject to close his eyes.
4. Separates the two pointed ends of a divider 2-3 cm apart.
5. Randomly touches one or both ends on the affected part.
6. Asks the subject to inform when the divider is felt.
7. Reports correctly.

PROCEDURE STATION-9

Demonstrate the procedure of testing stereognosis in the subject provided.

Checklist

1. Instructs the subject.
2. Makes him comfortable.
3. Asks the subject to close his eyes.
4. Gives him familiar objects to feel.
5. Gives more than one object.
6. Asks subject to identify the object.
7. Reports correctly.

QUESTION STATION

1. What is a tactile aesthesiometer used for?
2. How is deep pain tested?
3. What is hyperalgesia?
4. How is sensory ataxia different from cerebellar ataxia?
5. Name two diseases in which vibration sense is lost?
6. What is the name given to loss of stereognosis? Where is the site of damage?
7. What is paresthesia?
8. Draw a flow diagram showing the pathways for crude touch, pain and vibration sense?

Chapter 54

Clinical Examination of the Visual Acquity

PROCEDURE STATION

Demonstrate the procedure of testing visual acquity of the subject.

Checklist

1. Instructs the subject.
2. Makes him comfortable.
3. Seats subject at appropriate distance from the Snellen's chart.
4. Checks that lighting is adequate.
5. Asks the subject to close the other eye.
6. Makes the subject read from the top to the bottom.
7. Alternately make him read in between letters for conformation.
8. Tests both eyes.
9. Reports correctly.

QUESTION STATION

1. Define the term visual acquity?
2. What is normal visual acquity expressed as?
3. What is myopia?
4. What is hypermetropia?
5. What is the nature of lens used in spectacles of a myopic?
6. Name the chart used to check near vision?
7. What rule must be followed while making the Snellen's chart?
8. At what distance must a subject sit from the snellens chart for measurement of his visual acquity?
9. How will you test visual acquity in a child?
10. How will you test visual acquity in an illiterate person?

Clinical Examination of the Visual Acquity 119

11. A subject can read upto the third line from above in the Snellen's chart
    a. At what distance from the subject is the chart normally kept?
    b. What is the visual acquity of the subject?
    c. Name one physiological and one pathological factor which can affect the visual acquity?
12. Identify the chart.

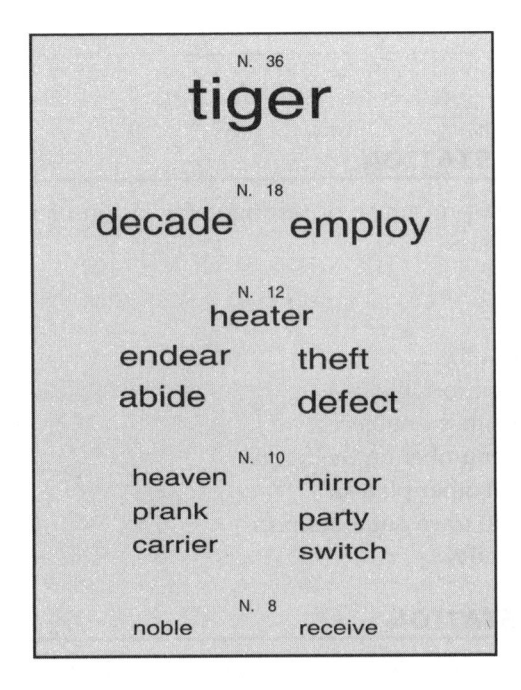

```
              N. 36
            tiger

              N. 18
        decade    employ

              N. 12
              heater
        endear      theft
        abide       defect

              N. 10
        heaven      mirror
        prank       party
        carrier     switch

              N. 8
        noble       receive
```

Chapter 55
Clinical Examination of Color Vision

PROCEDURE STATION

Demonstrate the procedure of testing color vision of the subject using Ishihara chart plates.

Checklist

1. Instructs the subject.
2. Makes him comfortable.
3. Shows a plate to the subject.
4. Asks him the number on the figure.
5. Moves over to other plates.
6. Asks subject to trace out a design.
7. Reports correctly.

QUESTION STATION

1. In which professions is color vision testing mandatory?
2. Name the various procedures for testing color vision?
3. What is the physiological basis of colors used in the Ishihara plates?
4. How will you test for color vision in an illiterate person?
5. What is the most common color blindness reported?
6. What is the genetic basis of color blindness?

Chapter 56
Clinical Examination of the Eye by Retinoscopy and Ophthalmoscopy

PROCEDURE STATION
It is avoided as pupillary dilatation is required.

QUESTION STATION
1. Identify the instrument (Ophthalmoscope or retinoscope).

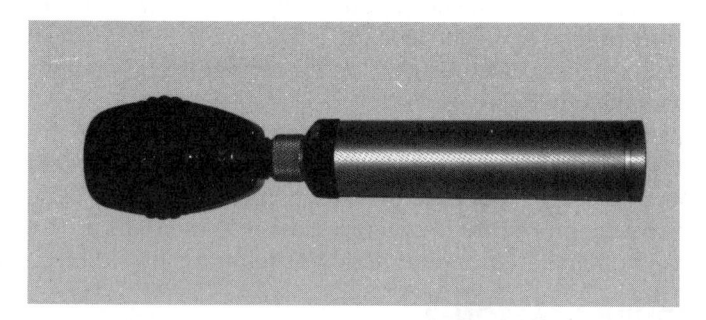

2. What is the type of mirror used in a retinoscope?
3. What is observed during a normal retinoscopic examination?
4. Name the type of disorder if the image moves on the same side as the reflecting mirror in the retinoscope?
5. Name the type of disorder if the image moves on the opposite side compared to the reflecting mirror in the retinoscope?
6. Besides the refractive state what other information can the retinoscopic examination provide?
7. What is the type of mirror present in an ophthalmoscope?
8. What all can be observed with an ophthalmoscope?
9. What is the difference in the working and the image formed in direct and indirect ophthalmoscope?
10. Draw a diagram to show the appearance of the normal optic disc using a direct ophthalmoscopy?

Chapter 57

Examination of Field of Vision by Perimetry

PROCEDURE STATION-1

Demonstrate the procedure of mapping the field of vision by perimetry.

Checklist

1. Instructs the subject.
2. Makes him sit comfortably in front of the apparatus with the chin in the appropriate chin rest.
3. Adjusts the level of the head of the subject so that the lower lid of the eye touches the tip of the leveling bar.
4. Asks the subject to fix his gaze on the central fixation point.
5. Covers the other eye.
6. Adjusts the metallic arc and moves the target with a rod.
7. Notes and marks the point when the subject sees the target first.
8. Moves the target spot upto the fixation point to look to blindspot.
9. Repeats the procedure in other meridians at intervals of 15 degree.
10. Joins the points in different meridians to map the field of vision.

PROCEDURE STATION-2

Demonstrate the procedure of mapping the blind spot by perimetry.

Checklist

1. Instructs the subject.
2. Makes him sit comfortably in front of the apparatus with the chin in the appropriate chin rest.
3. Adjusts the level of the head of the subject so that the lower lid of the eye touches the tip of the leveling bar.
4. Asks the subject to fix his gaze on the central fixation point.
5. Covers the other eye.
6. Adjusts the metallic arc in the horizontal plane in the temporal quadrant.
7. Moves the target with a rod.
8. Notes and marks the point when the subject sees the target first.
9. Moves the target spot up to the fixation point.

10. Marks the point when the target disappears to reappear again.
11. Joins the two points when the target is visible in a circular line.
12. Labels the blind spot.

PROCEDURE STATION-3

Demonstrate the procedure of mapping the field of vision by confrontation.

Checklist

1. Instructs the subject.
2. Makes him sit comfortably facing the observer, 1 metre away.
3. Asks the patient to look into the observer's eyes.
4. The tip of finger is moved in each of the four quadrants (superotemporal, superonasal, inferotemporal, inferonasal.
5. Asks the patient to report when he sees the object.
6. Reports correctly.

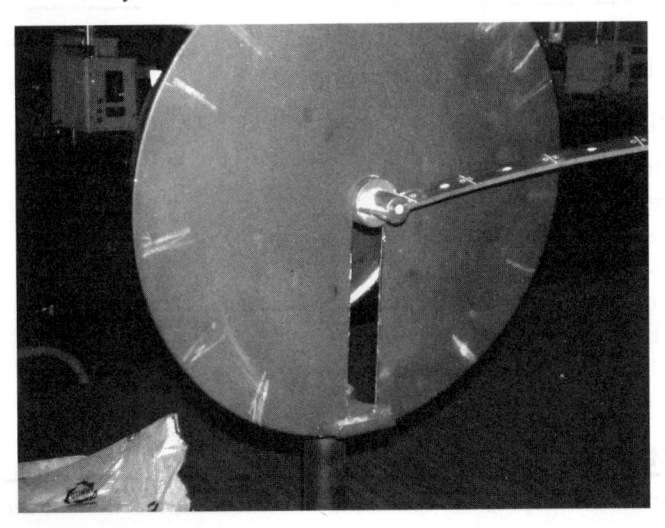

QUESTION STATION

1. Identify the instrument. What is it used for?
2. A perimeter chart is provided to you. Comment on the field of vision marked in the chart?
3. What is the normal extent of field of monocular vision and binocular vision?
4. What is the blind spot? On which side of the field of vision is the blind sot presence. What does it represent?
5. Name a physiological and a pathological condition that can limit the field of vision?
6. How does size and color affect the field of vision?

Chapter 58

Clinical Examination of Cranial Nerves

Testing visual acuity, color vision is also important for the second cranial nerve. Similarly, the test for hearing is important for the eighth cranial nerve.

PROCEDURE STATION-1

Demonstrate the procedure of testing the first cranial nerve in the subject provided.

Checklist

1. Instructs the subject.
2. Makes him comfortable.
3. Tests each nostril separately.
4. Chooses the right testing material.
5. Applies or bring it near the nostril to be tested.
6. Asks the subject to identify the smell.
7. Tests the other nostril after some time.
8. Reports correctly.

PROCEDURE STATION-2

Demonstrate the procedure of testing the direct light reflex on the subject provided.

Checklist

1. Instructs the subject properly.
2. Positions the subject according to the light source.
3. Positions himself properly.
4. Separates the eyes or closes the eye not tested (light not to reach it).
5. Asks the subject to look at a distant object.
6. Brings torch from the side.
7. Shines it in the eye to be tested.
8. Looks for the constriction in the pupil.
9. Removes the light immediately.
10. Looks for pupillary dilatation.

PROCEDURE STATION-3

Demonstrate the procedure of testing the consensual light reflex on the subject provided.

Checklist

1. Instructs the subject properly.
2. Positions the subject according to the light source.
3. Positions himself properly.
4. Separates the eyes or closes the eye not tested (light not to reach it).
5. Asks the subject to look at a distant object.
6. Brings torch from the side.
7. Shines it in the eye to be tested.
8. Looks for the constriction of the pupil in the other eye.
9. Removes the light immediately.
10. Looks for pupillary dilatation.

PROCEDURE STATION-4

Demonstrate the procedure of testing the third cranial nerve of the subject provided.

Checklist

1. Instructs the subject properly.
2. Checks each eye separately.
3. Asks the subject to follow movement of his hand.
4. Moves his fingers upwards from the horizontal position.
5. Moves his fingers towards the medial direction.
6. Reports correctly.

PROCEDURE STATION-5

Demonstrate the procedure of testing the fourth cranial nerve of the subject provided.

Checklist

1. Instructs the subject properly.
2. Checks each eye separately.
3. Asks the subject to follow movement of his hand.
4. Moves his fingers downwards and outwards from the horizontal position.
5. Reports correctly.

PROCEDURE STATION-6

Demonstrate the procedure of testing the sixth cranial nerve of the subject provided.

Checklist

1. Instructs the subject properly.
2. Checks each eye separately.
3. Asks the subject to follow movement of his hand.
4. Moves his fingers laterally from the horizontal position.
5. Reports correctly.

PROCEDURE STATION-7

Demonstrate the procedure of testing the facial nerve of the subject provided.

Checklist

1. Instructs the subject properly.
2. Asks the subject to inflate cheeks.
3. Taps on the cheeks.
4. Asks the subject to whistle.
5. Asks the subject to show his teeth.
6. Tries to look for other signs (facial symmetry, expression, nasolabial fold, angle of mouth, eyebrow position).

PROCEDURE STATION-8

Demonstrate the procedure of testing the ninth cranial nerve of the subject provided

Checklist

1. Instructs the subject properly.
2. Makes him comfortable.
3. Takes a substance to be tested.
4. Puts it on the back of the tongue.
5. Tickles the back of the pharynx with a swab stick.
6. Looks for the gag reflex or asks the subject to write down the taste.
7. Reports correctly.

PROCEDURE STATION-9

Demonstrate the procedure of testing the tenth cranial nerve of the subject provided.

Checklist

1. Instructs the subject properly.
2. Makes him comfortable.
3. Asks the subject to say "Ah."
4. Looks for movements of both sides of the palatal arch.
5. Reports correctly.

PROCEDURE STATION-10

Demonstrate the procedure for testing the eleventh cranial nerve

Checklist

1. Instructs the subject properly.
2. Moves the chin on one side against resistance.
3. Looks for drooping of the shoulders.
4. Shrugs the shoulders against resistance.
5. Performs on both sides.

PROCEDURE STATION-11

Demonstrate the procedure of testing the twelfth cranial nerve of the subject provided.

Checklist

1. Instructs the subject properly.
2. Makes him comfortable.
3. Asks the subject to protrude out his tongue.
4. Asks the subject to move his tongue from side to side and lick each cheek.
5. Reports correctly.

Chapter 59
Clinical Examination of Hearing

PROCEDURE STATION-1

Demonstrate the procedure of doing the Rinne's test on the subject provided.

Checklist

1. Instructs the subject properly.
2. Positions of the examiner is appropriate.
3. Holds the tuning fork properly.
4. Strikes it properly.
5. Keeps the vibrating tuning fork on the mastoid process of the patient.
6. When he stops hearing, brings tuning fork next to the patient's ear.
7. Keeps the Tuning Fork parallel to the ear.
8. Asks subject whether he can hear or not.
9. Reports correctly.

PROCEDURE STATION-2

Demonstrate the procedure of doing the Weber's test on the subject provided.

Checklist

1. Instructs the subject properly.
2. Positions of the examiner is appropriate.
3. Holds the tuning fork properly.
4. Strikes it properly.
5. Keeps the vibrating tuning fork on the vertex, chin, midline of the patient.
6. Positions the tuning fork appropriately.
7. Asks subject whether he can hear equally or not in both ears.
8. Reports correctly.

PROCEDURE STATION-3

Demonstrate the procedure of doing the Schwabach's test on the subject provided.

Checklist

1. Instructs the subject properly.
2. Positions of the examiner is appropriate.
3. Holds the tuning fork properly.
4. Strikes it properly.
5. Keeps the vibrating tuning fork on the mastoid process of the patient.
6. Positions the tuning fork appropriately.
7. Asks subject whether he can hear, and raise his finger when he no longer can.
8. Places the tuning fork on his own mastoid process to check.
9. Reports correctly.

PROCEDURE STATION-4

Demonstrate the procedure of testing positional sense on the subject provided.

Checklist

1. Instructs the subject (Keep eyes open, report vertigo).
2. Makes him comfortable.
3. Seats the subject on the examination couch.
4. The subject back is straight.
5. The subject head is turned 45 degree on left/right.
6. The subject is lowered 30 degree from the horizontal level (Maintain this position for 20 - 30 seconds).
7. Looks for nystagmus.
8. Repeats with the head turned in the opposite side.

PROCEDURE STATION-5

Demonstrate the procedure of testing middle ear disease by the fistula test on the subject provided.

Checklist

1. Instructs the subject.
2. Seats him comfortably.
3. Presses the tragus into the internal meatus.
4. Uses a speculum/pneumatic bulb to push in air in the ear.
5. Reports correctly.

PROCEDURE STATION-6

Demonstrate the procedure of testing vestibular function on the subject provided.

Checklist

1. Instructs the subject.
2. Makes him stand with feet together.
3. Makes him stand with arms outstretched.
4. Makes him stand with eyes open and then closed.
5. Reports correctly.

PROCEDURE STATION-7

Demonstrate the procedure of testing oculocephalic reflex on the subject provided.

Checklist

1. Instructs the subject.
2. Keeps him supine.
3. Holds his head in both hands.
4. Keeps the eyes open with the help of the two thumbs.
5. Rocks the head briskly from side to side.
6. Notes the movement of the eyes (normal response eyes move in opposite direction to the head).

QUESTION STATION

1. Besides clinical examination, name other tests that provide information of the auditory system?
2. Name the tests routinely done to test the vestibular function?
3. Name two causes of conductive, sensorineural deafness?
4. Name two causes of otorrhea?

Chapter 60
Clinical Examination of the Motor System

PROCEDURE STATION-1

Demonstrate the procedure of testing the coordination in the upper limb on the subject provided.

Checklist

1. Instructs the subject properly.
2. Asks the subject to touch his nose bringing his hand from the lateral side.
3. Places his finger so that the patient touches examiner's finger and his own nose.
4. Performs with eye closed.
5. Tests for adiadokinesia.
6. Reports correctly.

PROCEDURE STATION-2

Demonstrate the procedure of testing the coordination in the lower limb on the subject provided.

Checklist

1. Instructs the subject properly.
2. Exposes the leg till above the knee.
3. Asks the subject to move his heel of the other foot from the knee downward.
4. Asks the subject to move in a straight line.
5. Observes Rhomberg sign with eyes open and closed.
6. Reports correctly.

PROCEDURE STATION-3

Demonstrate the procedure of testing the motor system of the right upper limb subject.

Checklist

1. Checks the bulk of the muscles.
2. Checks the tone of the muscles.
3. Compares with the other limb.
4. Checks for the strength of the muscles of hand, forearm and upper arm.
5. Checks for coordination by performing the finger nose test and ask the subject to make circles in the air.
6. Reports correctly.

PROCEDURE STATION-4

Demonstrate the procedure of testing strength of the forearm muscle.

Checklist

1. Makes the subject comfortable.
2. Places the forearm of the subject in midprone position and asks him to flex against resistance.
3. Places the forearm against the chest and asks him to straighten it out against resistance.
4. Places the subjects hand in full supination and asks him to flex against resistance.
5. Compares with the other limb.
6. If there is any weakness detected in any of above, and then check the grade by doing movement against gravity, with gravity, flicker of movement.
7. Reports correctly.

PROCEDURE STATION-5

Demonstrate the procedure of testing rebound phenomenon.

Checklist

1. Makes the subject comfortable.
2. Asks the subject to stretch out his arms in front and maintain this position.
3. Pushes the patient's wrist quickly downward and observe the returning movement.

PROCEDURE STATION-6

Demonstrate the procedure of testing rapid alternating movements.

Checklist

1. Makes the subject comfortable.
2. Demonstrates the act of repeatedly patting the palm of one hand with the palm and the back of the other, as quickly and regularly as possible.
3. Asks the subject to copy/repeat your actions.
4. Repeats with the other hand.

PROCEDURE STATION-7

Demonstrate the procedure of testing gait of the subject.

Checklist

1. Asks the patient to walk about 10 metres, turn around 180° and return.
2. Notes the time taken.
3. Notes the length, width of steps and tendency to sway.
4. Asks the patient to walk heel to toe in a straight line.
5. Looks for gait instability.
6. Reports correctly (hemiplegic's gait with circumduction, bilateral UMN damage-scissor like stance, cerebellar dysfunction- broad based gait, Parkinson's disease-short shuffling gait, festinant gait, proximal muscle weakness-waddling gait, Bizarre-Psychogenic).

PROCEDURE STATION-8

Demonstrate the procedure of meningeal irritation of the subject.

Checklist

1. Instructs the subject.
2. Makes him lie supine with no pillows.
3. Makes him lie without pillows.
4. Exposes both legs.
5. Fully extend both legs.
6. Supports the subjects head with fingers at occiput, ulnar border of hand next to paraspinal muscles of the neck.
7. Flexes the neck gently to touch the chin on the chest.
8. Flexes one leg at the hip and knee joint.
9. Supports this position with hand placed on the hamstring.
10. With the other hand extends the knee.
11. Looks at the patient for sign of pain, winching, or flexion of the other leg as a reflex.
12. Reports correctly.

QUESTION STATION

1. Name one condition when the following may be found:
   a. Wasted muscle.
   b. Hypotonia.
   c. Rigidity.
   d. Sensory ataxia.
   e. Irregular heel knee test.
   f. Babinski positive sign.
   g. Abnormal babainski rising up sign.
   h. Dysdiadochokinsia.
   i. Drunken gait.
   j. Festinant gait.
   k. Intention tremor.

Chapter 61
Clinical Examination of Higher Functions

PROCEDURE STATION

Demonstrate the procedure of testing the higher functions of the subject provided.

Checklist

1. Makes the patient comfortable.
2. Asks about the date, month, and time of the day.
3. Asks him small mathematical problems.
4. Tells the patient a name.
5. Asks him to repeat it, immediately and after 5 minutes.
6. Tells him a word.
7. Asks the subject to write it down.
8. Writes a word on the paper.
9. Asks him to say out.
10. Reports orientation to time and place, intelligence, memory and speech.

QUESTION STATION

1. Define delusion and hallucination?
2. What is the difference between dementia and depression?
3. What is the standard method of testing intelligence in a subject?
4. What is the etiological difference between loss of recent and long term memory?
5. Assign a diagnosis:
    a. A person is unable to understand spoken word
    b. A person is unable to understand written word
    c. A person is unable to speak
    d. A person is unable to write
    e. A person's speech is slow
    f. A person is unable to speek more than 2-3 words
    g. A person talks excessively, but speech makes little sense.
6. Differentiate between aphasia and dysarthria?
7. What is global aphasia and global amnesia?
8. What do you understand by the term coma?

Chapter 62
Clinical Examination of Reflexes

PROCEDURE STATION-1

Demonstrate the procedure of eliciting the knee jerk on the subject provided.

Check list

1. Explains the procedure to the subject.
2. Exposes the part to be examined.
3. Positions the subject appropriately.
4. Holds the hammer properly.
5. Strikes it properly.
6. Strikes it at the proper site.
7. The jerk is elicited.
8. If not tries Jendrassik's maneuver.

PROCEDURE STATION-2

Demonstrate the procedure of eliciting the biceps jerk on the subject provided.

Checklist

1. Explains the procedure to the subject.
2. Exposes the part to be examined.
3. Positions the subject appropriately.
4. Holds the hammer properly.
5. Strikes it properly.
6. Strikes it at the proper site.
7. The jerk is elicited.
8. If not tries Jendrassik's maneuver.

PROCEDURE STATION-3

Demonstrate the procedure of eliciting the triceps jerk on the subject provided.

Check list

1. Explains the procedure to the subject.
2. Exposes the part to be examined.
3. Positions the subject appropriately.
4. Holds the hammer properly.
5. Strikes it properly.
6. Strikes it at the proper site.
7. The jerk is elicited.
8. If not tries Jendrassik's maneuver.

PROCEDURE STATION-4

Demonstrate the procedure of eliciting the ankle jerk on the subject provided.

Checklist

1. Explains the procedure to the subject.
2. Exposes the part to be examined.
3. Positions the subject appropriately.
4. Holds the hammer properly.
5. Strikes it properly.
6. Strikes it at the proper site.
7. The jerk is elicited.
8. If not tries Jendrassik's maneuver.

PROCEDURE STATION-5

Demonstrate the procedure of eliciting the planter jerk on the subject provided.

Checklist

1. Explains the procedure to the subject.
2. Exposes the part to be examined.
3. Positions the subject appropriately.
4. Uses an appropriate object.
5. Uses it properly.
6. Uses it in the proper direction.
7. The jerk is elicited.

PROCEDURE STATION-6

Demonstrate the procedure of eliciting the abdominal jerk on the subject provided.

Checklist

1. Explains the procedure to the subject.
2. Exposes the part to be examined.
3. Positions the subject supine.
4. Uses an orange stick to stroke briskly.
5. Moves in a medial direction across the upper and the lower quadrants of the abdomen.

PROCEDURE STATION-7

Demonstrate the procedure of eliciting the Hoffman jerk on the subject provided.

Checklist

1. Explains the procedure to the subject.
2. Exposes the part to be examined.
3. Places the right index finger under the distal interphalangeal joint of the patient's middle finger.
4. Flicks the patient's finger downward with the right thumb.
5. Looks for reflex flexion of the patients thumb.

PROCEDURE STATION-8

Demonstrate the procedure of eliciting the finger jerk on the subject provided.

Checklist

1. Explains the procedure to the subject.
2. Exposes the part to be examined.
3. Places his index and middle finger across the palmar surface of the patient's proximal phalanges.
4. Taps his own fingers with a hammer.
5. Observes for flexion of patients fingers.

QUESTION STATION

1. Define spinal shock?
2. Name the stages of shock?
3. What is the physiological basis of Jendrassik's maneuver?
4. What is the importance of knowing which reflex is absent/exaggerated?
5. Write the grading of reflex?
6. Name each reflex and give the root values of the nerves involved?

Chapter 63

Determination of Reaction Time

PROCEDURE STATION-1

Demonstrate the procedure of recording the visual reaction time of the subject provided (circuit is already made for the student).

Checklist

1. Checks the circuit.
2. Instructs the subject to release his key as soon as the bulb glows.
3. Moves the drum at maximum speed.
4. Records a straight line on the drum with a signal marker.
5. Asks the subject to press his key.
6. Now presses his keys to complete the circuit such that the bulb glows.
7. Takes a time tracing.
8. Calculates the visual reaction time.

PROCEDURE STATION-2

Demonstrate the procedure of recording the auditory reaction time of the subject provided.

Checklist

1. Checks the circuit.
2. Instructs the subject to release his key as soon as he hears the tapping of the key.
3. Moves the drum at maximum speed.
4. Records a straight line on the drum with a signal marker.
5. Asks the subject to press his key.
6. Now presses his keys to produce a tapping noise.
7. Takes a time tracing.
8. Calculates the auditory reaction time.

QUESTION STATION

1. Define reaction time and reflex time?
2. What is choice reaction time?
3. Give the normal value of the visual reaction time?
4. Give the normal value of the auditory reaction time?
5. Name two factors that can decrease the reaction times?
6. Name two factors that can increase the auditory reaction time?

Chapter 64

Electroencephalography

QUESTION STATION

1. Identify the instrument/picture of the instrument placed in front. What is it used for?

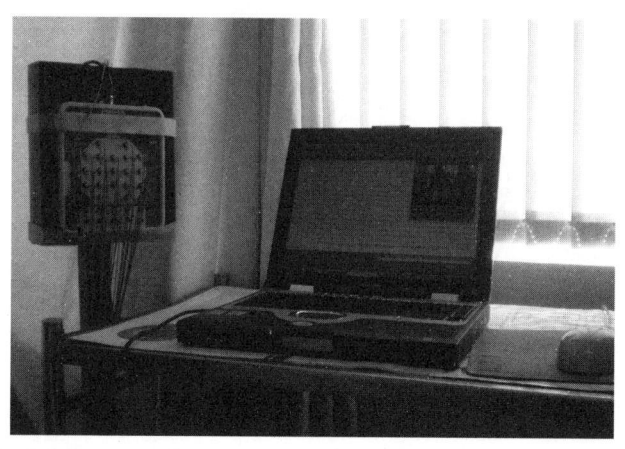

2. Identify the tracing/record. What information can be obtained from it?

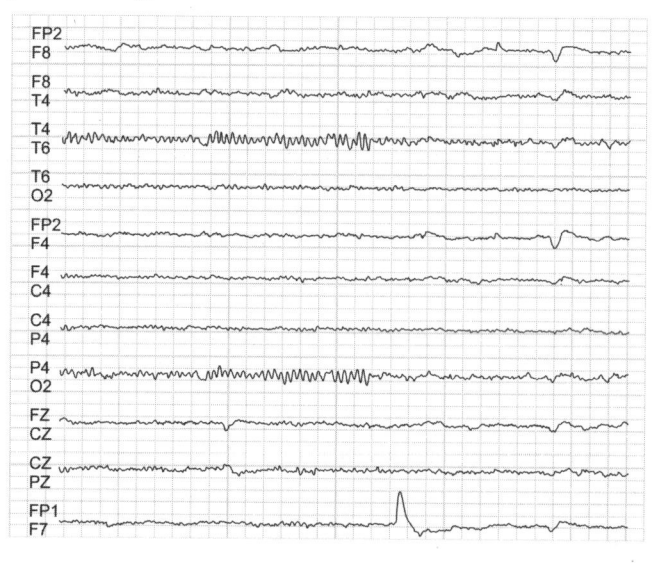

3. What is an electrocorticogram?
4. Name the common waves obtained with an EEG. Write down their frequency and the site where they prefentially occur?
5. What do you understand by the term "synchronization"?
6. Name two factors which increase and two which decrease synchronization?
7. What is "alpha block"?
8. Name two diseases where the above investigation is essential for diagnosis?

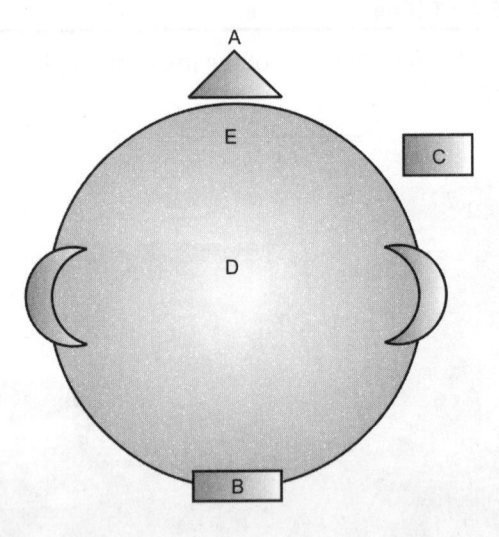

9. On the diagram given, label the landmarks (diagram of 10 - 20 system, labeled is to be provided)?

Chapter 65

Evoked Potentials

QUESTION STATION

1. What are evoked potentials? How are they different from EEG?
2. Name the waves recorded from an auditory brainstem response?
3. Name the waves recorded from a visual evoked response?
4. What is an event related potential?
5. In the diagram given, mark the waves labeled?

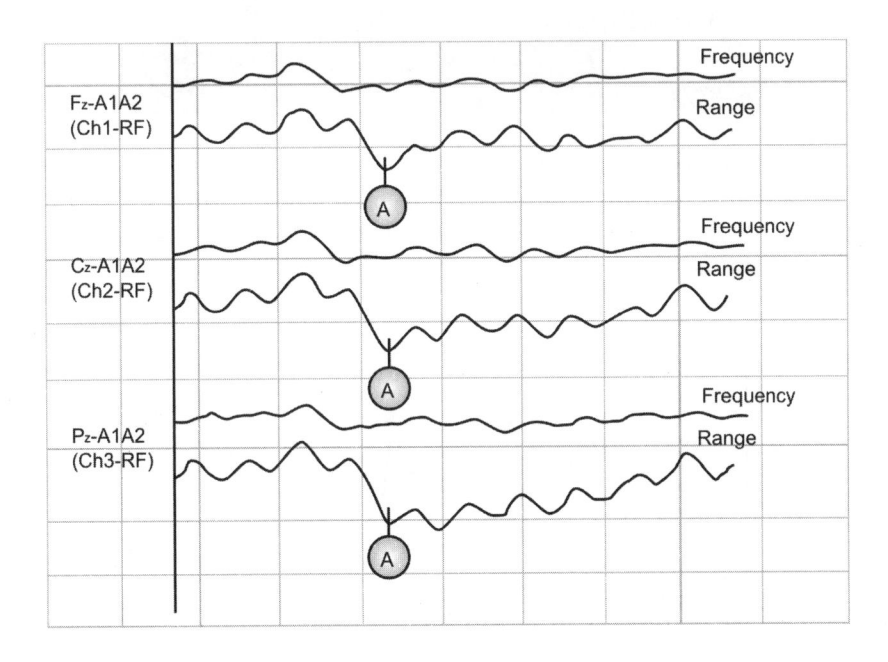

6. What is the cause of delay in latency of P300 wave?
7. In an ABR response what does the interpeak latency I-V signify?
8. The apparatus shown is used to record an important physiological variable?

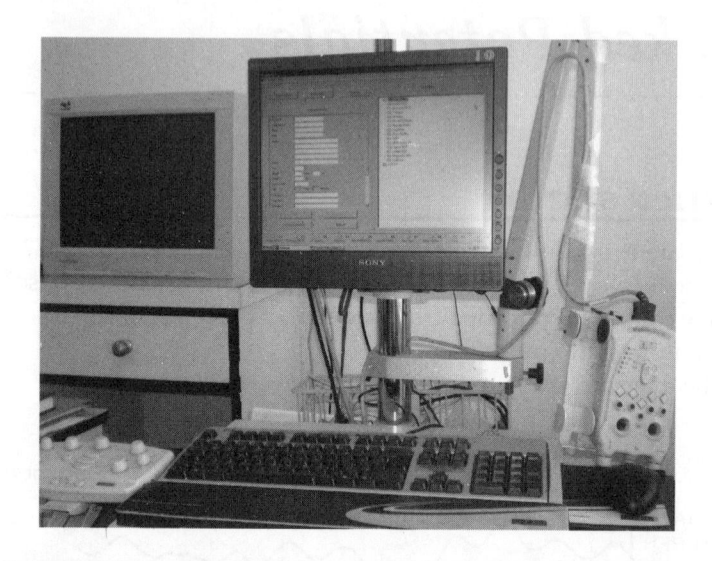

   a. Identify the apparatus?
   b. Describe the main features of the recording obtained?
   c. Enumerate four clinical conditions that can be diagnosed using the apparatus?
9. Identify
   a.

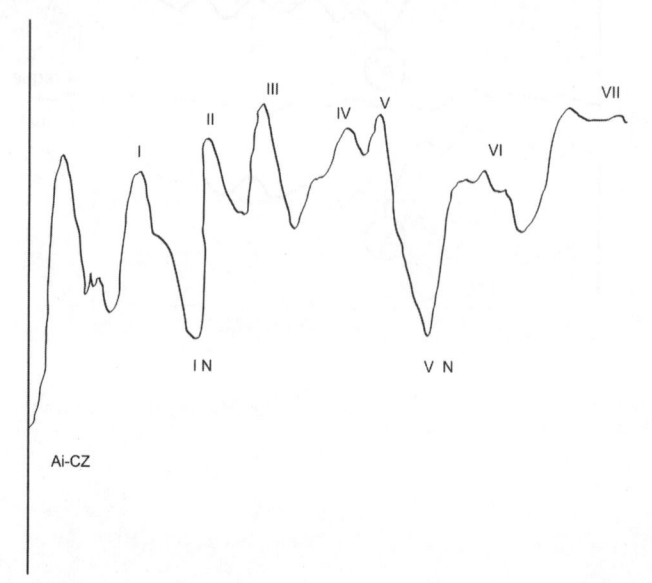

b.

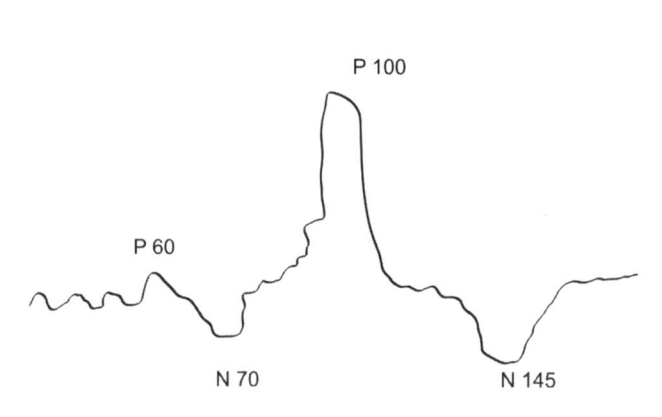

P 100

P 60

N 70   N 145

10 g retinal
Luminance
=2.86

Pupil
natural

Answers

The question stations and their probable answers are mentioned. There cannot be an ideal answer and the answers may vary with minor alterations in the questions.

Unit 1: Hematology

Study of Compound Microscope

1. This is a compound microscope.
2. Depending upon the part marked.
3. Compound and electron microscope.
4. a) 40X ;   b)100X
5. Oil immersion.

Collection of Blood Sample

1. Ethylene diamine tetra-acetic acid and trisodium citrate.
2. Heparin
3. a. EDTA is used as a sodium or a potassium salt which acts as a chelating agent for calcium in blood.
   b. Trisodium citrate: This forms an insoluble salt with calcium.
   c. Heparin: It facilitates the action of antithrombin III. Hence, the active form of factor IX-XII will be inhibited and coagulation will not take place.
4. Needle enters in first attempt, does not prick the doctor. Blood does not spill.
5. Hepatitis B, AIDS.

Specific Gravity

1. a. Depends on the experimental set up.
   b. It is heavier than the solution.
   c. It is lighter than the solution.
   d. Hammer Schlag method/direct method.
   e. It gives an idea about the cellular, molecular and water content of blood.
2. a. Subject to diagram.
   b. Yes (generally for physiology OSPE).
   c. Physiological conditions like pregnancy and pathological condition like dehydration.

Answers

3. a. No.
   b. Indirect and direct method. Indirect copper sulphate method.
   c. Gives us an idea about the concentration of cellular and water content of blood.

Hemoglobin

1. a. 1.34 × 16 = Oxygen carrying capacity.
   b. 3.34 mg × 16 = Iron content.
2. Calorimetry, Haldanes method.
3. Fetal hemoglobin, oxyhemoglobin, methemoglobin.
4. Acid hematin.
5. a. N/10 HCl.
   b. This method is standardized for HCl in a particular concentration.
   c. Hemoglobin present in the blood reacts with the N/10 HCl to form acid hematin. This value is standardized.
6. a. New born, high altitude.
   b. Blood quantity is not accurate, fading of comparator plates.
   c. 1.34 ml × 20.
7. a. Subject to experiment.
   b. Calorimetry.
   c. Male 14 - 18 gm%, 23 - 12.5 gm% depending from birth to one year.
8. a. Estimating hemoglobin.
   b. Level to decrease compared to standard.
9. a. Packed cell volume or peripheral smear examination.
   b. It is microscopic hypochromic anemia.

RBC Count

1. a. Subject to experiment.
   b. About 7μ
   c. Less number of RBC and increase in pallor.
2. 400 × 10, 000 = 4 million per cubic mm.
3. Dilution factor = final volume of solution/original volume of blood
   = 100/0.5
   = 200 times.
4. Subject to experiment
5. Tells us about the functioning of bone marrow and erythropoiesis, anemia.
6. Autoanalyzer.
7. RBC count and Hb estimation.
8. *Less no* of RBC, Increase in central halo of RBC. If treatment is adequate than the above defect is corrected plus there is increase in reticulocyte count if done.

9. Caliber and marking of the tube first and the red bead.
10. If the RBC count decreases markedly then it can be used.
11. Subject to experiment.
12. MCV.
13. RBC pipette: (a) RBC count (b) characteristic marking.

RBC Indices

1. a. $45/5 = 90 \ \mu m^3$
   b. MCH, MCHC.
   c. Important for morphological classification of anemia.
2. a. MCHC = Hb in gm × 100/PCV per 100 ml of blood.
   Amount of hemoglobin expressed as a percentage of the volume of RBC or hemoglobin concentration in one RBC.
   b. Hb and PCV.
   c. Peripheral blood smear, the size of RBC appears smaller and they appear pale (increased central pallor).

Osmotic Fragility

1. (a) and (b) subject to experimental condition.
   (c) Mechanical fragility.
2. 5 % glucose isotonic.
3. 0.9 % saline.
   5 % glucose
4. Normal breakdown of RBC and increased breakdown due to drugs.
5. a. Within normal limits.
   b. Increased.
   c. Sodium citrate, double oxalate.
6. a. It is decreased (normal range 0.48 - 0.34)
   b. Drugs and infection.
7. a. 0.48 - 0.34
   b. Spherocytosis (Increased)
   Sickle shaped anemia (decreased)
   c. 1% sodium chloride solution
   d. When the concentration of saline becomes less than 0.9 %(isotonic), saline enters the RBC due to osmosis and the RBC will burst. When the lysis begins it is called onset of fragility.
8. Written above.

ESR and PCV

1. a. Wintrobes and westergrens
   b. For measuring ESR.
   c. Westergrens preferred. A longer tube is more accurate.

Answers

2. a. Wintrobes tube.
   b. 0 - 9 in males and 0 - 20 in females.
   c. PCV.
3. a. Normal;
   b. Any infection or tissue damage.
   c. The cells settle down when left for some time as their density is greater than that of plasma. In one hour most of the cells >95% settle down. Any change which affects the surface area, density of cell or the viscosity of the plasma may alter the settling rate.
4. a. The lowermost layer of RBC, the buffy layer in between consisting of WBC and the platelets, the clear plasma above.
   b. The PCV increases.
   c. The cellular and water content of the blood and its variations.
5. a. It is 40 - 50% with an average of 45%.
   b. It gives us an idea of RBC count. If WBC, platelet increases, buffy coat is more
   c. If the red cells count increases leading to polycythemia because of hypoxia at high altitude, then the PCV will increase.
6. a. It is high.
   b. Infection/Anemia/Malignancy.
   c. Venous blood is mixed with sodium citrate solution. 3.8% to prevent coagulation. It is sucked up into the Westergren's tube till mark 0. The upper end of the tube is closed to prevent the blood from flowing out. Now it is fixed vertically in a wooden stand and the cells allowed settling down due to rouleaux formation.
7. a. Either wintrobe or westergrens.
   b. As in (a)
   c. Ratio of cell to plasma; viscosity of plasma.
8. a. Subject to experiment.
   b. With the passage of time the value will increase.
   c. 4 - 7 mm in the first hour (westergren)
      0 - 20 (wintrobe)
9. a. Subject to experiment
   b. Westergren's is more sensitive
   c. Already written.

Blood Group

1, 2 subject to blood provided.
3. a. All can donate blood provided they are Rh +ve
   b. Direct crossmatching and observation of vitals during transfusion.
4. a. Nil in both cases
   b. Nil
5. a. Not much reaction.

b. O -ve.
   c. Land Steiner's law.
   d. Anti B.
6. a. Anti A.
   b. IgM
   c. IgG
7. a. No.
   b. O+ve, AB +ve, A+ve, B +ve.
   c. Written above.

Reticulocyte Count

1. a. Reticulocyte
   b. 1% brilliant cresyl blue in isotonic saline.
   c. < 2%
2. a. Staining under living conditions at 37°C. This is required for the RNA to take up the stain.
   b. The cells (ribosome) take up the stain in living conditions when all the transport mechanisms across the cell are operating appropriately.
   c. The blood mixed with the stain is to be kept in an incubator at 37°C for 15 - 20 min to enable the stain to enter the cell. The smear prepared from this is neither fixed nor counterstained.
3. a. Hb level, reticuloyte count.
   b. Reticulocytosis occurs first.
4. a. It is a vital stain the cells are living.
   b. I. 0.2 - 2%;
      II 2 - 6%.
   c. To check the bone marrow response to treatment.
5. a. Reticulocyte.
   b. Size slightly bigger than the surrounding RBC, blue stain, reticulo-filamentous material present in the cytoplasm.
   c. Vital staining.

Total Leukocyte Count

1. N × 50.
2. 10/0.5=20 dilution factor.
   4×0.1 mm^3 = n
   1 mm^3 = n/0.4
   1 mm^3 = n/4 × 10 × 20 (dilution factor)
   = 50 n (multiplication factor)
3. TLC, DLC.
4. < 11000
5. *Turks fluid:* RBC cannot be visualized glacial acetic acid lyses the membrane and there is no nuclei which can be stained.

Answers

6. a. As per experiment.
   b. Done above.
   c. Proper filling of pipette and charging of chamber.
   Rule of counting should be followed and the same cell should not be counted twice.

Differential Leukocyte Count

1. a. Increase in eosinophils and leukocytes.
2. Normal.
3. Eosinophils increased.
4. As per experiment.
5. As per experiment.
6. Number, size and hemoglobin content of the RBC. WBC: number and size and differential count, platelets adequate, presence of parasite, lead poisoning, etc.
7. pH = 6.8, It causes ionization of the stain so that it can enter the cell.
8. Leishman's and Wright's stain.
9. a. The blood smear fixes on to the slide. It cannot be washed off. It maintains the cells in the state (chemical/metabolic); they were in before the onset of the experiment.
   b. Acetone free methyl alcohol.
   c. Acetone can cause shrinkage of and crenation and even lysis of the cell.
10. a. Written above.
    b. The granules are large course, red in color and do not obscure the nucleus.
    c. *Clinical value:* Relative number of RBC, WBC and platelet. To diagnose-type of anemia, DLC for acute, chronic infection and parasitic infection.
11. a. Eosinophils are high.
    b. Allergic or parasitic infection.
12. a), b), c), e) are subject to experiment.
    d. Leishman's stain.
13. a. Subject to experiment.
    b. Size <2/3, lines not continuous, gaps, thick, thin.
    c. 2 and 8 minutes for stain and buffered water.

Eosinophil Count

1. a. Subject to experiment.
   b. DLC and TLC.
   c. Pilot's stain.
2. a. Eosinophil
   b. Size of the cell, bilobed nucleus and big, red coarse granules.

c. The granules contain enzymes and chemicals which help to carry out the function (Major basic protein, eosinophil, cationic protein, histaminase peroxidase.
3. a. The WBC squares.
   b. Subject to data provided.
   c. Allergic reactions.
4. a. 50 n
   b. Pilots solution.
   c. The pilots solution contains phloxine which stains the eosinophil granules, propylene glycol, a solvent which lysis the RBC, sodium carbonate which lysis other RBC and heparin an anticoagulant.
5. a. Eosinophil
   b. Bilobed nucleus, coarse red granules in cytoplasm.
   c. I. Worm infestation
      II. Bone marrow depression.
6. a. Eosinophil % high
   b. Absolute eosinophil count, stool examination.
   c. Recruitment of eosinophils at the site as a protective mechanism.
7. a. Subject to data provided.
   b. Written above.
   c. Granules are coarse and red. They are lysosomal and may contain larvicidal or other enzymes that help to limit infection.
8. a. Subject to data provided.
   b. Pilots
   c. Absolute: Actual increase in eosinophil number. Relative—the % of eosinophil has increased. It could be because of the decrease in the number of other cells.

Bleeding and Clotting Time

1. a. Yes.
   b. If increased indicates a deficit in coagulation mechanism of blood.
   c. Platelets function to maintain homeostasis by affecting capillary integrity which affects bleeding time. If the coagulation factors are present the clotting time will not be affected.
2. a. Capillary tube method. Lee and white method.
   b. The presence of clotting factors, platelet factor and their activity. Calcium and temperature.
   c. The time for conversion of prothrombin to thrombin under experimental conditions. It is about 11 - 23 seconds depending upon the lab standardisation.
   d. I. *Clotting time:* The exact time must be noted. The capillary tube should be broken frequently but small pieces at a time.
      II. *Bleeding time:* The time of onset of bleeding must be correctly noted. Do not press too hard on the blotting paper.

Answers

3. a. Yes.
   b. *Bleeding time 2 - 6 minutes:* Clotting time 2 - 8 minutes.
   c. All these investigations are carried out at 37°C. If the temperature is decreased the vessel wall is constricted and the bleeding time will decrease. Similarly clotting time requires the activity of enzymes which function well at body temp and whose kinetics is affected by the temperature.
4. a), b) Subject to the data provided.
   c. Purpura (bleeding time), Christmas disease (clotting time)
5. a), b) Subject to experimental conditions.
   c. Lee white method.

Platelet Count

1. a. It is a colorless solution so other bottles containing pilot's, Leishman's may be provided also.
   b. *Diagram of platelets:* Only low power observations.
   c. 1.5 - 5 lac/mm^3
2. a. Subject to diagram provided.
   b. Implies that the chamber has not been charged properly.
   c. 2000 n
3. a. 2 - 5 minutes.
   b. Platelets are destroyed in the spleen. Its removal means more availability in the circulation which may to decrease in both the times.
   c. Hemostasis, clot retracton.
4. a. Platelet count.
   b. Factor VIII
   c. *Hess test or sphygmomanometer test:* A cuff is tied on the upper arm and the pressure is raised in-between the systolic and the diastolic blood pressure. This impedes the venous outflow, allows arterial flow and thereby increases the pressure in the capillaries. If fragile they will give way leading to petechie in the cubital fossa. A positive test occurs when the petechiae are more than 20 in an area of 3 cm diameter in the cubital fossa.

Bone Marrow Examination

All questions depend on the slides provided.

Unit 2: Amphibian Experiments

Simple Muscle Twitch

1. Subject to graph provided. Find out the time period between the point of stimulus and point of contraction. Each contraction of the 100Hz tuning fork corresponds to a time of 0.01 sec.
2. Temperature, frequency of stimulation. An increase in the temperature and frequency of stimulation will fasten the reaction and decrease the latent period.
3. Contraction period from point of contraction till maximum height. Relaxation period from the maximum height till point of relaxation. If the second stimulus is given in this period the response varies. Also in the fatigue experiment the relaxation will be incomplete.
4. Approximately 0.1 sec
5. So that the exact point of stimulus can be marked.
6. Isotonic.
7. The action potential is drawn in the beginning of the contraction phase. It can be shown divided into the absolute and the relative contraction period.
8. Tetanizing frequency = 1/contraction period (in millisecond).
9. Depending on whether it is a free or an after loaded condition. In after loaded condition the height of contraction decreases, in freeloaded condition the work output may increase up to the optimum load. A load lengthens the latent period decreases the contraction and the relaxation period, height of contraction.
10. Sciatic nerve and gastrocnemius muscle.
11. When the strength of the stimulus is increased, more motor units are recruited and the height of contraction increases.
12. It can be changed by changing the distance between the primary and the secondary coil.
13. The height of contraction correlates with the distance moved to lift the load. Hence, it can give an idea about the work done.
14. The relaxation period is slightly longer. Only 0.01 sec. The reason could be mechanical friction or otherwise.
15. It has 0.6% NaCl, 0.14 % KCl, 0.012% $CaCl_2$ and 0.02%$NaHCO_3$.
16. *Cold blooded animal:* Temperature maintenance and direct oxygen supply not needed.
17. Suprathreshold stimulus preferred so that maximum number of motor units are recruited.
18. Entry of sodium during depolarization and efflux of potassium during repolarization.

Answers

19. In the contraction phase there is conductance of sodium and potassium. Release of calcium from the sarcoplasmic reticulum. In relaxation calcium is pumped back into the sarcoplasmic reticulum. Calcium released from troponin.
20. Subject to experimental setting.

Effect of Temperature on Simple Muscle Twitch

1. When hot ringer is added the rate of contraction is increased, all the time periods decrease, force of contraction increases. For cold ringer the opposite effect takesplace.
2. As per record.
3. Above 45° denaturation of enzymes will take place.
4. Mentioned above.
5. Muscle activity is best in the normal body temperature range.
6. Various phases are slowed.
7. Denaturation of proteins. No proper graph appears.

Effect of Two Successive Stimuli on SMT

1. a. A; b) Supramaximal to eliminate the effect of beneficial effect on the strength of stimulus; c) Latent period. d) Some calcium availability remains to increase the force of contraction.
2. a. Subject to experiment; b) See diagram.
3. a), b), See original experiment. c) The response due the second stimulus is more. This is due to availability of ions.
4. a. The two prongs of the striker are separated so that two stimuli are delivered when the contact with the kymograph is established.
   b. Yes to identify the point of stimulus.
   c. See diagram.
5. As per experimental setup.

Effect of Increasing Strength of Stimulus

1. By decreasing the distance between primary and secondary coil.
2. Faradic break shock.
3. As the strength of currant s increased more and more motor units are recruited and the response measured by the height of contraction increases. A stage is reached when current is supramaximal, all motor units are recruited and further increase in strength of current produces no additional response.
4. Subthreshold refers to the strength of current below that required to illicit a response.
5. A motor neuron with all the musle fibres it supplies constitutes a motor unit.

6. Threshold stimulus is that which will illicit response. In maximal stimulus all motor units will be recruited.
7. Yes, each muscle fibre obeys this law.
8. The strength of any muscle contraction increases with the strength of stimulus.

Effect of Increasing Frequency of Stimulus

1. A–treppe; B–clonus; C–Incomplete tetanus; D–Complete tetanus.
2. *A and B:* In A there is complete relaxation, not seen in B; in B and C–the frequency of stimulus is more in C, so the period of relaxation decreases.; In C and D–In D there is no relaxation at all.
3. Neef's hammer and Variable interrupter.
4. *Twitch duration:* The time taken for a simple muscle twitch to occur.
   Tetanising frequency: The frequency of stimulus necessary to produce tetanus.
   Summation: The addition of current strength, stimulus or response. Generally availability of ions is increased.
   Tetany: A state of hypeerexcitability of skeletal muscle characterized by decrease in serum calcium levels.
5. Cannot be tetanised because it has a long refractory period. Second stimulus will fall in the refractory period.
6. Unnecessary stimulation of the preparation in-between the recording to be avoided. Neef's hammer and the variable interrupter to be connected separately.
7. Approx 74 times.
8. Muscles maintaining posture remain in a state of tetanus.
9. Yes as above.
10. *Contracture:* In this the muscles are in a state of contraction. The ATP is depleted and relaxation is thus not possible as it requires ATP. Reversible.
    Rigor: Extreme rigidity. Depletion of ATP hence phosphocreatinine. If after death called rigor mortis. Irreversible.
11. See diagrams.
12. Explained above.
13. As per experimental setup.
14. a b c d e
15. a) and b) Means the same. When second stimulus is given in the relaxation phase of the first, the tension developed in each twitch increases and height of contraction increases.
16. Fatigue—Depletion of neurotransmitter.
17. Calcium availability decreases. All events occur earlier.
18. Tetanus will not occur.

Answers

After Loaded and Free Loaded Condition

1. A—Free loaded. Moving drum
   B—After loaded. Moving drum
   C—After loaded. Static drum
   D—Free loaded. Static drum.
2. *Free loaded:* Load acts on the muscle before it begins to contract.
   After loaded: Load acts on the muscle after the contraction has begun.
3. *After loaded:* Lifting weight from the ground.
   Free loaded: Continuous contraction of the antigravity muscle.
4. Work done = Force × Distance = 20 g × 20 × L × 981 ergs.
5. Formula for distance move by the lever= height of contraction × l/L, where l is the distance between the fulcrum and the load and L is the distance between the fulcrum and point of writing lever.
6. Optimal load refers to that where maximum work is done.
7. Optimal length is the length of the muscle when it is lying at rest in the body in natural conditions. At this length the muscle is capable of developing maximum active tension.
8. Optimal length.
9. Yes, Preload is the freeload acting on the heart or cardiac muscle before it begins contraction. This load will stretch the muscle increasing the initial length, hence force of contraction. After load is the resistance which acts on the muscle after it starts contracting. It refers to the resistance in the outflow of blood from the left ventricle. Could be due to valvular defect of the aorta, Aortic stenosis.
10. As per experimental conditions.
11. W = Force × distance = weight lifted in grams × 981 × l/L × H where l is the distance between the fulcrum and the load and L is the distance between the fulcrum and point of writing lever. H is the height of contraction.
12. As above.
13. In free loaded condition the muscle is already stretched. The number of cross linkages between actin and myosin is less. So contraction is earlier, more work can be done. Force of contraction is more.
14. Work one will increase till the optimum load and then decrease. Equilibrium length- it is the length of muscle when it is cut from its attachment to the bones. Resting length—it is the length of the muscle when it is lying in the body in its natural environment.
15. Written before.
16. *Written before:* An after loaded condition is created by connecting the after loaded screw. It creates a mechanical situation that prevents the weights from acting on the muscle or stretching it at rest. Once the contraction begins the force of the weights will act on the muscle.
17. As per experimental conditions.

Fatigue

1. *Fatigue:* A temporary reduction in the working of a muscle which may be reversed after renewal of supplies of nutrients, oxygen etc.
2. The increase is due to beneficial effect of repeated stimulation. Then decrease occurs due to causes that lead to fatigue.
3. *Neuromuscular junction:* Muscle is not the site of fatigue. Direct stimulation of the muscle produces a contraction. With the help of ice block preparation, it can be proved that the nerve is not the site of fatigue.
4. Central/CNS.
5. If you flex your wrist, any muscle for long, it will start paining.
6. Depletion of nutrients and oxygen.
7. Tetanus involves a sustained contraction of the muscle but in a fatigue contraction of muscle will not occur.
8. By intermediate relaxation of the muscle, massaging etc.
9. There is increase in enzymatic activity, mitochondria, recruitment of capillaries, so the work capacity increases. Fatigue is delayed compared to a sedentary person.
10. 1- first contraction; 2, 3-beneficial effect; 70-fatigue (no relaxation); DS-direct stimulation showing that muscle is not the site of fatigue.
11. a. As above; b) Ice block experiment.
12. As above.
13. a), b) as above; c) depletion of neurotransmitter.
14. a. Increasing weight lifted, delay in conducting the experiment.
    b. Fatigue is reversible if depleted stores of nutrients, O_2 and neurotransmitter are replenished.

Isometric Contraction

1. *Isotonic contraction:* When the muscle is stimulated the tension increases, to maintain which the muscle contracts thereby decreasing its length. Isometric contraction—here the length of the muscle is kept constant, so there is increase in tension.
2. Isometric lever is used. Calibrated before.
3. More external work will be done when there is movement/ shortening as in isotonic.
4. *Isotonic:* Walking; isometric—posture maintaining muscles.
5. *Active tension:* The difference between total and passive tension is the tension due to contraction, called active tension. It refers to the tension in the contractile processes.
   Passive tension is the tension exerted by the unstimulated muscle and varies with the length of the muscle.

Answers

Conduction Velocity of Sciatic Nerve

1. A vertebral end; B muscle end.
2. Muscle end-faster conduction, less loss of tension, so height of contraction is more.
3. The latent period is different because one stimulus (vertebral end) has to traverse the entire length of the nerve to stimulate the muscle.
4. Two stimulators are connected to the secondary key. One group stimulates each end of the nerve supplying the muscle.
5. Distance between the two ends of the nerve/ time (difference in the latent periods).
6. The difference in the latent periods of the two contractions has to be found.
7. Median/ulnar nerve.
8. Calipers are used to find the length of the nerve in-between the two ends.
9. Aα 70 - 120 m/s; Aδ 12 - 30 m/s; C 0.5 - 2 m/s.
10. Decrease in temperature, fatigue.
11. The conduction velocity can be increase by increasing the temperature, alteration of contents of the conducting media.
12. a. As per experimental conditions;
    b. Temperature, diameter of the nerve fiber, myelination, closeness of RMP to threshold of stimulation.
13. a. As per experimental condition;
    b. On the basis of function, diameter and hence conduction velocity differs.
14. Lesser latent period is the muscle end. Increased diameter and myelination leads to more conduction velocity.
15. a. 2 sets of stimulating electrodes to be used.
    b. By an oscilloscope, electrodes placed at the elbow for stimulation of the ulnar nerve. Recording electrodes at the wrist.
    c. It tells you about the type of nerve fiber. In injury/ trauma the nerve may be damaged leading to an increase in velocity. As recovery occurs it comes back to normal
16. As per experimental condition.

Normal Cardiogram and Effect of Temperature

1. a) In 5 sec - 7; in 60 sec - 7 × 60/5 = 84/min.
2. 20 - 30 beats/min;
3. a) Atrial systole, b) Atrial diastole; c) Ventricular systole; d) Ventricular diastole.
4. Signal marker.
5. *Human:* SA node; frog- sinus venoses.
6. Autorhymicity

7. *Downsroke:* As per arrangement of the ventricle, pin and lever, when ventricle contracts it pulls the lever down.
8. 2.5 mm/sec.
9. Sinus venosus, 2 atria and 1 ventricle.
10. Do not puncture, injure the ventricle; prevent the cardiac tissue from drying.
11. Warm ringer increases the heart rate and force of contraction. The opposite occurs for the cold ringer.
12. In fever heart rate increases.
13. Yes, except for the anatomical arrangement, the functioning is identical, O_2 may be required for the human heart.
14. The function is similar, no O_2 is required. Temperature maintenance is not necessary.
15. In isolated heart, ringer has to be continuously supplied. In intact heart the effect of neurotransmitter added may be modified by others present.
16. As above.
17. As per experimental conditions.

Properties of Cardiac Muscle

1. Heart block, All or none law.
2. By mechanical pressure, stannous ligature.
3. Show cardiac activity followed by a straight line (no activity).
4. Thoractomy, atriotomy and ligation of AV bundle. Injection of chemical through a transvenous catheter into node or AV bundle.
5. It returns but the other areas may take over.
6. See text.
7. Ist stannous ligature-sins venoses and atria; 2nd stannous ligature atrio-ventricular groove, atria and ventricle.
8. The first returns quickly within minutes. The second idioventricular rhythm may take up to one hour.
9. Idioventricular rhythm 6 - 12 beats per minute.
10. It may last long enough to cut off oxygen to the brain.
11. As per experimental conditions.
12. When an extra stimulus is give when the heart is in diastole there may be an extra-premature contraction, called an extrasystole. So in the normal graph a response is achieved earlier. After that there is a compensatory pause (Straight line).
13. Ectopics.
14. A series of subthreshold stimuli given (Shown by recording of the signal marker) ultimately produces a response.
15. Minimal stimuli also affect the heart. If frequent, may add to produce a response.

Answers

16. A—Extrasystole, B—Compensatory pause.
17. A-First stannious ligature; B-second stannious ligature; C-Idioventricular rhythm.
18. All or none law.
19. Summation of subminimal stimuli.
20. a) Sinus rhythm; b) Yes functional syncytium.
21. a) Autorhythmicity; heart block, extrasystole and compensatory pause, Effect of temperature, all or none law, summation of subminimal stimuli, staircase phenomenon, effect of drugs, effect of vagal stimulation. b) All or none law; Staircase phenomenon; Summation of subliminal stimuli.
22. a) Same height contraction; b) Functional syncitium; c) Written before.
23. a, b, as per diagram, of beneficial effect, all or none law.
24. a) 6 - 12-beats per minute; b) proper tying of ligature, no external injury, proper idioventricular rhythm to establish; c) about 0.5 hour.
25. a, b, c, d, h.
26. b, e.
27. A cardiac cycle.

Effect of Vagal Stimulation

1. Graph A—vagal stimuli, cardiac activity inhibited, graph B—vagal stimulation continued, C—vagal escape.
2. Both contain vagal fibers.
3. Below the platysma is the petrohyoid muscle. Over the shining tendon of levator scapulae lies the vagosympathetic trunk bundle. Vagus runs across this tendon as a white colored nerve.
4. Parasympathetic nerve fibers.
5. There is vagal escape. Contractility is again recorded. This is because the vagosympathetic trunk carries both types of fibers. Stimulation of vagus produces inhibition of the heart. Later the sympathetic nerve may be stimulated, neurotransmitter producing inhibition of heart may be reduced, or idioventricular rhythm may be established. These factors produce vagal escape.
6. Parasympatheic postganglionic fibers.
7. Atria have both sympathetic and parasympathetic supply via the T1-5 spinal segments and vagus response. The ventricles have only parasympathetic supply.
8. As above.
9. a) As above; b) Preganglionic cholinergic, postganglionicnoradrenergic.
10. a) Vagus; b) Parasympathetic fibres; c) Acetylcholine in both cases.
11. R1 preganglionic; R2 postganglionic. Acetylcholine.

Effect of Ions and Drugs on the Cardiac Muscle

1. Drug A is a stimulator, effect of vagus and WCL stimulation is preserved. Drug B slight stimulation. Drug blocks the vagus action. Drug C decreases effect. Effect of vagal stimulation is present.
2. Acetyl choline, low concentration of nicotine.
3. Adrenaline, atropine.
4. The drug decreases the cardiac activity. If given after atropine then no decrease in activity occurs.
5. The drug is stimulatory. When acetyl choline is given after the drug then the effect of acetyl choline is preserved.
6. In low doses the drug is inhibitory. Nicotine decrease cardiac activity by affecting vagus.
7. The drug may be slightly stimulatory. When acetyl choline is given after the drug then the effect of acetyl choline is not there.
8. Introduction of chemicals that destroy or block the vagus.
9. Drugs may act at receptors on the target organs. If this occurs then there will be no effect of vagus or WCL stimulation, but if only the ganglia are blocked then WCL (postganglionic fibers), produces effect. Vagus stimulation will be ineffective.
10. *Isolated heart:* No effect of milieu interior, no nervous connection.
11. *Mammalian heart:* Oxygen and temperature maintenance required.
12. By raising the tube/symes cannula, it increases the pressure of the fluid present.
13. NaCl⁻ No effect on heart rate. The force of contraction also shows minimal change. (may decrease) if Na competes with the Ca present.
14. It decreases both the heart rate and the force of contraction. If continued the heart may also stop in diastole.
15. No effect on heart rate, the force of contraction. Calcium rigor occurs with further calcium increase.
16. As per experiment.
17. As per experiment.
18. b, d, e, f, h.

Unit 3: Mammalian Experiments

Effect of Drugs and Ions on the Rabbits Intestine

1. Rabbit is a small mammal which can be conveniently handled.
2. Jejunum mainly.
3. Tyrode solution.
4. Tyrode contains 0.1 gm% glucose for nutrition, 0.8 gm% NaCl, 0.02 gm% KCl, and $CaCl_2$ each to provide the ionic and electrically balanced

Answers

solution, sodium bicarbonate and sodium dihydrogen phosphate to maintain pH. MgCl$_2$ may be added. Water is used to make the solution.
5. Mainly tonic and rhythmic movements. Peristaltic waves can also be demonstrated.
6. As per experiment.
7. Increased by acetylcholine and neostigmine; decreased by atropine and papavarine.

Effect of Drugs and Ions on the Rabbits Heart

1. Langendorff's apparatus.
2. Ringer Locke solution.
3. Mammalian preparation.
4. Yes
5. 7.1 - 7.6
6. Perfusion pressure is the pressure with which the solution flows through its path. It is about 60 - 80 mmHg. If it increases the fluid will enter the left ventricle leading to dilatation, if it is below then the preparation will fail to work after some time.
7. Increases both.
8. Langendorf's apparatus.
9. As per graph.
10. As the aorta is connected fluid enters it to pass on to the coronaries, to the myocardium, to the veins, the coronary veins, right atrium, superior and inferior venue cava and out. Some may enter the thebesian vein and into the left ventricle. And then the aorta.
11. Written above.
12. For adequate flow. Yes using a heart lung preparation. If the perfusion pressure is increased, stretching of the ventricles takes place increasing the force of contraction.
13. Adrenaline and acetylcholine.
14. Requirement of oxygen and maintenance of temperature.

Unit 4: Human Experiments

Mosso's Ergograph

1. a. Putting the BP cuff on the hand and raising the pressure in between the systolic and the diastolic BP. b) Work done is less in arterial occlusion as distance traveled is less. c) Motivation and replenishment of nutrition.

2. Q (graph Chap-29, page 61 and Chap-32, page 71)
   a. Wt × 980 × Distance
   $$\text{Distance} = \frac{\text{Area } (A - B) \times H + \tfrac{1}{2} B \times H^2}{A + B} \times \text{no: of contractions}$$
   b. 1) Neuromuscular junction, II) CNS.
3. a. Force × distance (Distance in detail)
   b. As above.
4. Mosso's ergograph. To show the phenomenon of fatigue in man.
5. To decrease the time of onset of fatigue.
6. Use timer or metronome.
7. By raising the BP in the cuff above the systolic BP.
8. Less work is done in arterial occlusion. Fatigue faster.
9. 10. Written above.
11. Depletion of neurotransmitter.
12. Yes.

Recording of Blood Pressure

2. Baroreflex.
3. Diastolic(60 - 80); systolic(100 - 120)
4. A period when no korotkov sounds are heard.
5. First the cuff is inflated, so as to occlude the artery. When BP is lowered a stage is reached when it matches the pressure during systole. The systolic BP is heard as the first audible sound on lowering the BP. A stage is reached when due to decrease in the external pressure the turbulence is decreased. The korotkov sounds become low pitched and muffled. This is the diastolic BP.

Effect of Posture on Blood Pressure

1. Systolic falls and diastolic increases or there is no change.

Effect of Exercise on Blood Pressure

1. In moderate exercise there is elevation in the heart rate, in the range 100 - 125, there is 25 - 50% of VO_2 max of oxygen consumption and 3 - 4.5 METS of energy used.
2. Systolic blood pressures is expected to increase. In untrained individuals diastolic BP may increase also.
3. Increase in sympathetic activity may bring about the effects.
4. Linear increase in blood pressure in moderate exercise. Only severe exercise suddenly may be harmful for patients. However, exercise has many long term benefits, in terms of cardiopulmonary fitness, muscle activity, metabolic activity. Regular exercise may cause reduction in hypertension.

Answers

5. Mild exercise increases systolic BP.
6. Severe exercise may increase both the systolic as well as the diastolic BP.

Plethysmography

1. Volume change per unit time.
2. Air tight chamber without leakage, float should be light, amount of muscle in forearm.
3. Doppler.
4. There is a specified range of blood flow to any organ. Increase in blood flow signifies vasodilation, increase blood supply, metabolic activity. Decrease in blood flow signifies vasoconstriction, localized obstruction, etc.

ECG

1, 2 as per ECG strip provided.
3. a. Electrocardiogram
   b. Calibration of equipment and earthing
   c. 25 mm/sec.
4, 5, diagrams.

Effect of Exercise on the Cardiovascular System

1. BP should be normal and the patient should not be having chest pain.
2. Weakness/fainting. Chest pain
3. Angina pectoris.
4. In all types of exercise the heart rate will increase with the severity of exercise. The systolic BP increases in all types exercise due to increase in cardiac output. Diastolic BP may increase only in severe exercise because of vasoconstriction in nonworking group of muscles and skin. In mild to moderate exercise there is vasodilatation in working group of muscles which leads to decrease in diastolic BP.
5. METS or metabolic equivalents are the multiple of the resting metabolic rate expressed as the oxygen uptake per minute per Kg. Usually resting metabolic rate is 3.5 ml/min/Kg average. For a 40-year-old 70 Kg man.
6. Tidal volume and rate of respiration will increase.

Study of Respiratory Movements by Stethography

1. a. These would be inspiration and expiration.
   b. It increases.
   c. *Cheyne-Stoke's breathing:* It is an abnormal pattern of breathing which develops slowly and is associated with alternate periods of apnea following hyperventilation.

2. a. Subject to graph provided.
   b. Inspiration and expiration.
   c. When the chest expands the length of the tube increases, since radius is constant, the change in length causes the change in pressure inside the tubing.
3. a. Stethograph.
   b. You can see movements of the chest wall and time them.
   c. It can tell you the effect of voluntarily controlling respiration by hyperventilation and breath holding on respiratory parameters like rate, force of ventilation. Gives an idea of certain reflexes.
4. a. Inspiration
   b. Hyperventilation causes carbon dioxide washout that causes an increase in the pH which is responsible for the apnea.
5. a. Inspiration is a down stroke. The time period of the straight line following the downstroke is to be calculated.
   b. Increase in oxygen intake, deep inspiration.
   c. Described above.
6. a, b, d, e described before. c) Breaking point. It is the point when breathing can no longer be voluntarily inhibited. It occurs due to fall of PO_2 and increase in PCO_2.
7. See diagram from standard text.

Spirometry

1 - 7. as per experimental condition.
8. >80% normal. Less in asthma.

Effect of Posture on Vital Capacity

1. *Vital capacity:* It is the maximum air that can be expired out following a maximum inspiration.
2. Standing.
3. Old age, kyphoscoliosis.
4. Males and athletes.

Effect of Exercise on Respiratory System

1. It increases due to increase in oxygen demand.
2. It increases. In moderate exercise it is due to increase in depth of respiration.
3. Blood lactate levels.

Measurement of Basal Metabolic Rate

1. For measuring resting metabolic rate by oxygen consumption.
2. Body and ambient temperature.

Answers

3. O_2 consumption/per minute= InitialO_2- Final O_2/time.
4. *Basal metabolic rate:* After a good nights sleep, 12 - 18 hours postabsorptive state, comfortable environmental temperature (20 - 25°C) and without any activity (moving), the oxygen consumption and thereby the metabolic rate is calculated, it is called BMR. It measures energy requirement for vital function. RMR measures the same after half an hours rest.
    b. Energy requirement for vital organs and maintain body temperature.
    c. Age, sex, diet, hormones etc.
5. a. 2 liters in 6 min; in 1 min 2000/6 ml.
    b. Corrected volume of oxygen consumed at STPD in 1 hr = 60 × 2000/ 6 × C (corrected volume at STPD)
    c. 1 liter of O_2 consumed per hr at STPD produces 4.875 k cal of heat at RQ 0.8; so heat produced=60 × 2000/6 × 4.875 × C.
6. a. Refer to age and sex normograms.
    b. Height and weight normogram.

Mechanical Efficiency

1. A steady state refers to that period during exercise when the O_2 consumption and the output become constant.
2. Work = Force × Distance;
    = 2 × 2000 Kgm
3. M.E = output/input × 100
    Output = 40 kilopond/min
    Input = 2.5 litres
    1 liter consumed gives aproximately 5 Kcal
    2.5 liter consumed gives 5 × 2.5 Kcal.
    426.7 Kpm/m= 1 Kilocal
    40 Kpm/m = 1/426.7 × 40 Kcal
    ME = output/input; 40/426.7X1/12.5 × 100 Kcal

Cardiopulmonary Resuscitation

1. Patency of the airways.
2. 12 - 16 breaths/min.
3. 70 - 80 beats/min. Ratio of resp/cardiac resuscitation =1:4 or 1:5
4. Mechanically pressing the chest wall.
5. Till help arrives or 30 minutes at least.
6. Chest size is small. Use thumb instead of full hand which is likely to cause damage. Also rate of massage will be faster.

Recording of Normal Body Temperature and Effect of Hot and Cold Environment on it

Semen Analysis

1. Count (80,000 - 120,000)/mm^3, 80% motile, normal morphology, opalescent, white color, 2-4 ml sample, pH 7.3 - 7.5.
2, 3) drawings.
4. Forward progressive motility.
5. Grade A- Fast progressive in a straight line.
   B—Slow progressive (slow linear or non linear motility)
   C—Non-progressive. Sperms move their tail but do not
   Move forward. (Local motility)
   D—immotile sperms.
6. Non-motile or local mobile sperms.

Pregnancy Diagnostic Tests

1. A—a
   B—b
   C—c
   D—d
2. a. HcG
   b. Choriocarcinoma
   c. 2 weeks in urine
   d. HcG
   e. > 25 mIU/ml.

General Physical Examination

CVS

1. a. Auscultatory areas.
      A—Aortic; B—Pulmonary; C—Tricuspid; D—Mitral area.
   b. S3 Third heart sound. Occurs due to filling of ventricles in early diastole.
      S3 is physiological in children and young adults and pregnancy. It disappears after the age of 40. It is low pitched, head with bell, after S2. S4 Fourth heart sound. Occurs due to filling of ventricles. It is generally heard as a low pitched, at the apex in LVH, hypertension, and aortic stenosis.
   c. Second heart sound during inspiration. P2 is delayed.
2. JVP a) Best seen with the patient reclining at 45°
   b. Arterial pulses are easily palpable, rhythmic, coinciding with the cardiac activity compared to the venous pulse.
   c. Congestive heart failure, Tricuspid valve disease.

Answers

Respiratory System

1. Vesicular breath sounds.
2. Asthma; chronic Bronchitis, rhonchi.
3. Midline or slightly to the right.
4. It is more delicate. So too much pressure should not be applied to the ribs.

Abdomen Examination

Sensory System

1. For tactile discrimination.
2. This is tested by squeezing the tendoachilles or the calf muscle.
3. Hyperalgesia is an exaggerated response to a painful stimulus.
4. Sensory ataxia. Is when the eyes are closed. In cerebellar ataxia, even with the eyes open there is ataxia.
5. Tabes dorsalis and peripheral neuropathies due to nutritional and metabolic causes.
6. Astereognosis. Parietal lobe.
7. Parasthesia refers to the presence of abnormal sensation.
8. See text.

Visual Acquity

1. Visual acquity is the degree to which the details and contours of the object are perceived. It is expressed in terms of the visual angle.
2. It is expressed as a fraction. The numerator is the distance at which an object stands/sits. = 6 meters. The denominator is the size of the letter. e.g. 24, 36, etc. This is the size such that at this distance, it subtends a visual angle of 5 minutes.
3. Refractive error with image formation in front of the retina.
4. Refractive error with image formation behind the retina.
5. Biconcave.
6. Jaeger's chart.
7. Size of letter must subtend a visual angle of 5 minutes at a particular distance. Width of letter, angle of 1 minute and interval distance between two lines, a distance of 1 min.
8. 6 meters.
9, 10. In infants visual acquity can be roughly assessed. Their eye movements are watched as rolling white balls of various sizes are placed in front of them. At 2.5 year or more Sheridan Gardiner test- The child/ his parent is made to hold a card with a number of letters on it. The examiner shows the child one letter and asks the child to point to the similar letter on the card. When the child has understood the test, the examiner moves to a distance of 6 meter from the child and shows

him a series of letters of decreasing size. The child matches on the card. This test is also useful in patients of dysphasia and in illiterate patients, or in those with a language problem. In Snellen's chart one option I the letter E or C, the patient is asked to point/tell which end is open, above, below, left or right.

11. a. 6 m.
    b. 6/24.
    c. Intensity of light in the room, myopia.

Color Vision

1. Drivers, pilots, surgeons, policemen.
2. Ishihara chart with pseudoisochromatic plates. Holmgrens wool, Edrige green lantern.
3. These plates are designed to identify people with color blindness. Numbers are presented in a series of colored dots, mixed such that it is not possible to make out the number for a color blind patient who may identify incorrectly or none at all.
4. Instead of numbers patterns are made with these colored dots. The patient is asked to trace the pattern with his/her finger on the chart.
5. It is red green blindness. Acquired defects of colored vision are seen in macula and optic nerve disease.
6. It is an X linked recessive condition.

Examination of Eye by Ophthalmoscope and Retinoscope

1. Ophthalmoscope or retinoscope will be provided.
2. Plane mirror.
3. A red glow with a black crescentric shadow its edge, is seen in normal individuals
4. This may be a normal vision, emmetropia, hypermetropia or myopia with less than one diopter.
5. Myopia.
6. The normal passage of light beginning from the cornea, when meets with any obstruction in its passage, it will appear as a black line against the normal reflex.
7. Concave and plane.
8. The retina, optic disc, macular, periphral region, blood vessels can be visualized. A larger image is obtained.
9. *Indirect*   *Direct*
   Examining distance of 1 metre   Closer to the patients eye
   Large concave mirror   Small concave mirror
   Magnified 5 times   Magnified much more.
10. Draw optic disc, in center, mark arteries, yellow and red appearing regions.

Perimetry

1. Perimeter for field of vision.
2. Subject to area marked.
3. *Monocular:* (Superior 60°, inferior 75°, Temporal 100°, medial 60°, Binocular 140° vertically, 200° laterally in the middle).
4. Blind spot is the area in the field of vision (temporal) where there is no perception of light. This represents the area on the optic disc where the optic nerve leaves the eye. There are no rods, cones (receptors) in this area.
5. Physiological—glasses, dim light. Pathological—Glaucoma, demyelination of optic nerve.
6. If the size of the object is increased, the field of vision is increased. Blue color has the largest field of vision followed by the yellow color.

Cranial Nerve

Tests of Hearing

1. Pure tone audiometry, speech audiometry, impedance audilogy, evoked response audiometry.
2. Eye movements, nystagmus, fistula test, Rhomberg sign, caloric test, rotational testing.
3. Conductive, ear wax, otitis media. Sensorineural, cochlea or retrocochlear pathology.
4. Acute otitis media and otitis externa.

Higher Functions

1. *Delusion:* A false belief in something that does not exist. Hallucinations- A false belief that something exists, pertaining to the sensory modalities of hearing, vision.
2. Dementia is a condition when the mental faculties decrease. Selective functions may be lost. It may progress over a time interval. Depression is on the other hand a psychiatric condition with neurochemical imbalance. The patient behaves in a dull manner. Corrected with drugs.
3. *IQ testing:* Alternatively standard questions, mathematical questions, application of knowledge, problem solving are used.
4. Recent memory, seconds to hours. Long term memory—Remote past. Different types of neurological disorders.
5. a. Anomic aphasia
   b. Anomic aphasia
   c. Motor aphasia
   d. Motor aphasia
   e. Motor aphasia

f. Motor aphasia
g. Sensory aphasia.
6. *Aphasia:* Defect in speech function, not due to motor paralysis, vision or hearing loss. Dysarthria is due to defect in motor area and connections. Difficulty in spoken speech. Muscles may be involved.
7. *Global Aphasia:* Defective speech due to involvement of both sensory (Wernick's) area and motor (Brocas) area. Global amnesia results in the loss of both recent and long term memory.
8. *Coma:* Refers to the state of a person when he/she makes no meaningful contact with the internal or external environmental condition.

Motor Examination

a. Muscle dystrophy
b. LMN lesion
c. Parkinsonism
d. Tabes dorsalis
e. Cerebellar ataxia
f. UMN lesion
g. Weakness of hip flexors and abdominal muscles
h. Cerebellar disease
i. Cerebellar disease
j. Parkinsonism
k. Cerebellar disease.

Reflexes

1. In an UMN lesion the initial stage of spinal shock is associated with loss of all reflexes.
2. Stage of spinal shock or flaccidity, followed by stage of reflex activity.
3. It increases the motor discharge and increases the excitability of the motor neurons. So, a better reflex is obtained. The subject may be distracted and less tense which may produce a more observable effect.
4. Gives an idea of the level of lesion. A LMN lesion will be observed at that level and a UMN below the level.
5. Grading 0—Absent; 1—Present (Intensity of the ankle reflex); 2—Brisk (intensity of the knee jerk); 3—very brisk; 4—Clonus.
6. *Superficial*—Scapular C5 - T1; Abdominal—T7 - 12; Cremastric L1 - 2; Plantar—L5 - S1; Anal S3 - S4; Conjunctiva, Corneal Cr5, 6, 7; Light reflex Cr2, 3; Palatial Cr5, 9, 10. *Deep*—Jaw jerk Cr5; Biceps, supinator C5 - 6; Triceps C6 - 7; Knee L2 - 4; Ankle S 1 - 2.

Answers

Reaction Time

1. Reaction time is the time interval between application of the stimulus and elicitation of voluntary response. Reflex time—It is the time interval between application of a stimulus and the initiation of an involuntary response.
2. *Choice reaction time:* This is the reaction time in a situation when there are two or more possible stimuli requiring different responses.
3. 200 - 400 msec.
4. 100 - 200 msec.
5. Practice, Attention.
6. Noise, sleep.

EEG

1. Electroencephalograph. For recording electrical activity of the brain. EEG.
2. Electroencephalogram. Different wave patterns are seen in different areas of the brain. These are compared to the normal in terms of frequency and the amplitude.
3. The record obtained when the electrodes are directly placed on the cortex.
4.

Wave	Frequency	Site
α	8-12	Parietooccipital
β	14-30	Frontal
λ	4-7	Parietal and temporal
δ	1-4	Sleep

5. The most common activity is the synchronized wave activity at rest with the eyes closed. Synchronization refers to the rhythmic pattern of electrical activity of one or more neighboring neurons.
6. Increased Synchronization—sleep and meditation. Decreased Synchronization in alertness and mathematical mental activity.
7. Blocking the rhythmic pattern. Replacing it with high frequency, irregular low amplitude activity/waves called the block.
8. Epilepsy, Brain tumor.
9. A—Nasion; B—Inion; C—Preauricular point; D—Vertex; E—frontal.

Evoked Potentials

1. Evoked potentials are potential differences recorded from the scalp in response to stimuli which may be visual, auditory or somatosensory. They are not present without stimulus.
2. Waves are labeled I- V. Other peaks are not of clinical interest. The latency and the interpeak latency are recorded.
3. The commonly used VEP are N70, P100, and N135. P represents a positive and N represents a negative wave.

4. When a subject has to pay attention to and voluntarily engage in activity such as counting nonverbally the number of stimuli, the potential recorded n the scalp are called event related potentials.
5. Subject to the diagram.
6. Deceased attention, neurological damage to an area.
7. Conduction delay from proximal 8th cranial nerve through pons to the midbrain.
8. a. Evoked potential machine.
   b. These are recordings of the potentials obtained from the scalp, when the subject is exposed to one or more stimuli. The response recorded is presented as waves. The amplitude, latency of theses gives an idea of the timing of conduction through the passage by various modalities.
   c. Neuropathy, demyelinating disorder, degenerating disorder, amnesia, cognitive disorder like Alzheimer's disease.

Index

A

Abdomen examination 171

B

Basal metabolic rate 91, 168
Bleeding and clotting time 30, 154
Blood group 19, 151
Blood pressure 73, 76, 77, 166
Body temperature 94, 170
Bone marrow 34, 155

C

Cardiac muscle 56, 162, 164
Cardiopulmonary resuscitation 93, 169
Cardiovascular system 83, 167
Clinical examination 171
    color vision 172
    cranial nerve 173
    eye 172
    hearing 173
    higher functions 173
    motor examination 174
    reaction time 175
    reflexes 174
    respiratory system 171
    sensory system 171
    visual acuity 171
Collection of blood 5, 148
Compound microscope 3, 148
Conduction velocity 161
Conduction velocity of the sciatic nerve 52

D

Differential leukocyte count 25, 153

E

ECG 81, 167
Electroencephalogram 175
Electroencephalography 141

Eosinophil count 28, 153
Erythrocyte sedimentation rate 16
ESR and PCV 150
Evoked potentials 175

F

Fatigue 49, 160
Free loaded condition 46, 159
Frequency stimulus 158
Frog's heart 61

G

General physical examination 99, 170
    abdomen 110
    cardiovascular system 103, 170
    color vision 120
    cranial nerves 124
    eye 121
    field of vision 122
    hearing 128
    higher functions 135
    motor system 131
    reaction time 139
    reflexes 136
    respiratory system 108
    sensory system 114
    visual acuity 118

H

Heart of rabbit 66, 165
Hemoglobin 8, 149

I

Intestine of rabbit 65, 164
Isometric contraction 51, 160

M

Mechanical efficiency 92, 169
Mosso's ergograph 71, 165

N

Normal cardiogram 54, 161

O

Ophthalmoscope 172
Ophthalmoscopy 121
Osmotic fragility 14, 150

P

Packed cell volume 16
Perimetry 122, 173
Platelet count 32, 155
Plethysmography 79, 167
Pregnancy diagnostic tests 98, 170

R

RBC count 149
RBC indices 13, 150
Red blood cell count 10
Respiratory movement 84, 167
Respiratory system 90, 168

Reticulocyte count 21, 152
Retinoscope 172
Retinoscopy 121

S

Sciatic nerve 161
Semen analysis 96
Simple muscle twitch 37, 39, 156, 157
Skeletal muscle contraction 40, 42, 43
Specific gravity 7, 148
Spirometry 87, 168
Stethography 84, 167
Strength of stimulus 157

T

Total leukocyte count 23, 152

V

Vagal stimulation 163
Vagus nerve white crescentic line 59
Vital capacity 89, 168